Little Something

Little Something

A Journey of Miracles From Infertility and IVF to Marathons and Motherhood

Elizabeth Lockwood

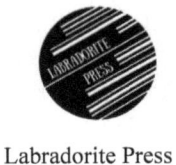

Labradorite Press

All rights reserved; no part of this book may be reproduced, stored in a retrieval system, or transmitted, in any form or by any means, without the prior permission in writing from the publisher, nor be otherwise circulated in any form of binding or cover other than that in which it is published and without a similar condition including this condition being imposed on the subsequent purchaser.

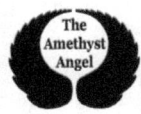

First published in Great Britain in 2018 by Labradorite Press, an imprint of The Amethyst Angel theamethystangel.com

Copyright © 2018 by Elizabeth Lockwood
Cover Design by The Amethyst Angel

ISBN: 978-1-912257-25-6

The moral right of the author has been asserted.

Every effort has been made to obtain the necessary permissions with reference to copyright material, both illustrative and quoted. We apologise for any omissions in this respect and will be pleased to make the appropriate acknowledgements in future editions.

Nothing in this book is to be taken as professional medical advice and is the opinion and experience of the author. The author and publisher accept no liability for damage of any nature resulting directly or indirectly from the application or use of any information contained within this book. Readers are advised to obtain medical advice before embarking on a fitness regime or diet, and any information acted upon from this book is at the reader's sole discretion and risk.

First Edition

For Tabitha

Contents

Chapter 1.	How it all began	1
Chapter 2.	How the hell am I going to do this?	15
Chapter 3.	Positivity, where are you?	25
Chapter 4.	When reproduction needs assistance	33
Chapter 5.	Run for your life	51
Chapter 6.	Give it one more go	61
Chapter 7.	When IVF fails	69
Chapter 8.	Rebuilding	79
Chapter 9.	Refocus	85
Chapter 10.	Finding strength	97
Chapter 11.	You must be crazy	107
Chapter 12.	Why don't you just adopt?	121
Chapter 13.	Acknowledge, accept, release	135
Chapter 14.	And then it all changed	141
Chapter 15.	Re(Birth)	153
Chapter 16.	Becoming a mother	163
Chapter 17.	New life	169
Chapter 18.	Motherhood is a strange beast	179
Chapter 19.	Why I believe in miracles	191
	Bibliography	197
	Acknowledgements	203
	About the Author	205

CHAPTER ONE
How it all began

My (in)fertility story began long before I could possibly have accurately predicted its outcome. I thought I knew what was going to happen many times, yet each time I was proved utterly wrong. As much as I like to plan everything, be organised and control things as much as possible, life has its own way of doing things and doesn't always want to conform to our meticulous plans. I learnt this lesson abundantly.

I was born in a small town in South Wales in the early 80s. My parents divorced when I was very young and my mother remarried when I was five. At the age of eight, my mum, stepfather, sister and I relocated, and that first move set the tone for a childhood of relocation, including spending three years in Toronto, Canada. I was an overweight child and found being funny or rebellious was a good way to defuse the relentless teasing. I was always a big dreamer, but struggled to bring any of those dreams into fruition due to deep insecurities. Despite hating school, I loved university and as a result never really wanted to leave. I studied English and gained three degrees. I met my husband when I was in the first year of my undergraduate degree at Aberystwyth

University, and not too long later we embarked upon our lives together.

For some reason, I had always thought that I wouldn't be able to have children. I'm not sure why. I didn't know anyone who was infertile, I wasn't aware of anyone around me experiencing infertility, it was just a thought that came and went intermittently at the back of my mind. The only reason I had to pay attention to those thoughts was the fact that I never had a regular menstrual cycle as described by doctors. And when I did, it certainly didn't seem 'normal' to me. I would often have extremely heavy bleeds and to me that somehow signalled that nothing worked in that area. I was a very self-conscious teenager, so it took a long time for me to build up the courage to visit the doctor to explain my symptoms. I was always obese, always had issues with cystic lesions on my skin and various other symptoms.

But despite going to the doctors from the age of sixteen it took until I was twenty-three for a doctor to finally join the dots and recognise that I had PCOS (polycystic ovary syndrome). During the many visits to various doctors previously I had repeatedly been told to go away and lose weight, a rather frustrating thing to say to a person who has been obese their entire life, seemingly regardless of food intake. I also felt like this was brushing aside and belittling my symptoms and experiences. It was as if I was being told to go away and stop faking. Like being told these symptoms meant nothing and it was my fault that I had all this trouble because I was fat and I had made myself that way. However, in January 2007, after finally finding a doctor who cottoned on to the situation immediately, I had all the required blood tests and scans and I received my diagnosis and an ongoing prescription for the drug Metformin.

My fiancé and I were due to get married later that year in

December, so we had to have a conversation about the possibility that I might not be able to get pregnant and whether or not he could accept potentially being unable to have our own children. We'd discussed having kids on and off in the past but never made any firm plans. After a while we'd both realised that we wanted children, but as we were in our early twenties at the time it didn't seem to be an urgent issue. However, now there was a sense of pressure surrounding the question, but despite this he was rather philosophical about the whole thing and said 'what will be will be', and we moved on with life and looked forward to our wedding. I started the medication and tried to lose some weight in the meantime. Clearly I didn't get very far as I got married without any weight loss and wasn't terribly bothered about it. We'd relocated and planned our wedding so it hadn't been my primary focus.

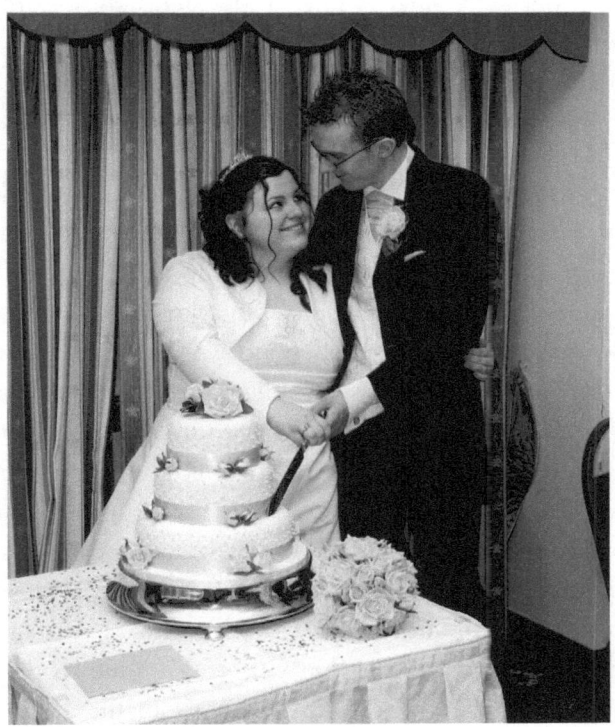

At our wedding (we were now both in our mid-twenties) I was surprised about how instantly the questions started – so, when are you going to have a baby then? I was about to start my research degree so I would divert the question and tell them I was too busy at the moment. But it was a nagging thought at the back of my head – could I even get pregnant? What would we do if we couldn't have any children?

After a lot of jokes about honeymoon babies and 'see you next at the christening' we forgot about these alcohol-fuelled comments and went off on our honeymoon. At that point pregnancy wasn't a common occurrence in the lives of those around me. We weren't that long out of university, so people were working on their careers and forming relationships. Pregnancy wasn't yet in everyone's horizons. Of course, not everyone wants children, and that's perfectly fine. Not everyone feels the desire or call to become a parent and they are happy with life as it is, with all the wonderful opportunities they can experience which do not involve having children in their lives.

A few months later in 2008, however, we decided that as it would likely be a struggle, or not even possible, for me to conceive, I would stop taking my progesterone only pill (the mini pill), as there seemed little point in bothering with it. It seemed like a sensible idea – if it was unlikely that I would fall pregnant easily, then why continue to take the pills? But almost immediately after stopping them, I started to get more involved in the idea of getting pregnant, despite the knowledge of my subfertility (reduced fertility). I would start looking for symptoms and doing tests each month just in case, because you never know... By the end of that year I was really starting to feel the frustration of being aware that my body just wasn't producing a pregnancy. I had even lost some weight that year (partly due to the weight loss drug Orlistat – but the least said about that drug and its oily urgency, the better), but unfortunately regained it when I plateaued at a certain point.

By 2009 I had developed that TTC (trying to conceive) obsession which many people experience – the 'why isn't it happening?' obsession. However, despite all those months without contraception, it still took until the very end of 2009 for us to decide we should visit the doctor to discuss it. I wasn't relishing going to see anyone – I didn't fancy another weight loss lecture and I didn't want to see my weight solely blamed for this problem. I already knew that losing weight would help my PCOS symptoms, but I just found trying to lose it so difficult. Whatever I tried, I seemed to get stuck at a certain point, a couple of stone lighter, and then become despondent and allow the weight to creep back on.

Despite being busy with university and work, I became completely obsessed with trying to get pregnant. The crushing disappointment each month (or longer than a month when my cycle disappeared randomly, causing false hope) when my period came, and the constant googling and reading forums and finding suggestions or ideas was becoming all-consuming. It seemingly started innocently enough… I'd join a forum, read posts, post questions, all perfectly normal things to do if you're hoping to get pregnant soon. But then one day you realise you've agonised over the potential positive (but clearly negative) pregnancy test and taken a photo of the test and posted it online for opinion. Not just that, somehow I ended up finding baby psychics online – I would pay for psychic readings and not one of them was anywhere near accurate. I can't comment on whether these people were just cashing in on the desperation of people wanting a baby or what – because maybe in some cases they were spot on – but the whole thing doesn't really sit right with me now. Anyone that markets themselves as providing readings for women trying to conceive specifically should probably be avoided. At this point in my life I wasn't really religious or spiritual, so I had no real idea of how to tell the good from the bad when it came to that sort of thing.

Month after month, I would somehow manage to half convince myself that I was pregnant – until my period came – and then I would be upset. How could this be possible? All the signs of pregnancy were there! Yes, that's one of nature's cruel little tricks – premenstrual symptoms and early pregnancy symptoms are quite similar. And if you're looking for signs, you'll quite often find them, even when they're not there. And it really wasn't just me; there were so many other women all agonising over the same stuff. All taking a photo of a faint line on a test and posting the photo on the forum, desperate to be told by faceless strangers that it was a line and not an evaporation line or no line at all. This seemed totally normal at the time. I know I'm making this sound like trying to get pregnant just turns you into a crazy person, but really, truly all of that is just a distraction from the heart breaking agony and bitter disappointment of wanting something you seemingly just cannot have.

Aside from dealing with the obsession side of analysing every little thing, there was also the issue of seeing pregnant women and babies everywhere. It seemed for a while that all I saw were pregnant bumps and prams, and even on social media it was nothing but scan photos and announcements. Initially it's exciting because you think, 'Ooh that'll be me soon! Can't wait!' and then slowly it starts turning sour, starts making your stomach hold onto a bit of resentment each time. This sourness hadn't quite developed into the extreme lows that I was to experience later on – at this point we still had some hope. Surely the doctor would sort us out? We'd get a prescription for something and be pregnant in no time. I'd read about it happening: one quick procedure to clean the tubes out or a month of pills and then there would be a baby.

Finally, at the end of 2009, we visited the doctor and while I'm sure weight was mentioned, he wasn't patronising at all, and agreed with us that despite weight, despite PCOS, if it hadn't happened in this time then it probably wasn't going to happen without some form of intervention. He referred us to a consultant at the hospital and we joined a waiting list of other subfertile couples holding onto the hope that the hospital would be able to sort things. I think we both felt sure that the consultant would be able to provide us with some form of treatment and we would at some point get pregnant, so when this referral was made it almost took some of the pressure off the situation.

Surprisingly, it wasn't a long time before we received our appointment letter for our initial consultation. One thing that I wasn't quite prepared for was the awkwardness of the infertility clinic. That initial appointment at the hospital was the first awkward experience of a long and tiresome awkward process. For some reason, they'd hold the infertility appointments at the same time as antenatal appointments, so you'd have heavily pregnant women in the same waiting room as women struggling to conceive. Talk about kicking you when you're down… I remember looking around at women with massive bumps and feeling like I was almost being mocked by the set up. Check it out – pregnant women! You're not pregnant, and you probably won't ever get pregnant! Then add in the awkwardness of people asking you when you're due and you have to tell them you're actually there for the infertility clinic.

My consultant was someone who was known for being a bit harsh and straight talking, but I didn't mind that. I wanted to know the facts and I could cope with being called out on my weight now – I'd heard it what felt like a million times before. I just didn't want my weight solely blamed as it had been so many times with my struggle for recognition of PCOS. So after that initial consultation we started with the preliminary tests. They wanted to confirm my PCOS again, which they did (unsure why – perhaps they thought I had just self-diagnosed through Google?). I had various blood tests, and my husband had the standard sperm analysis done.

I will admit that despite having smear tests in the past, this was a whole new experience of invasive vaginal examinations – internal scans, swabs, the lot. Including the HSG (hysterosalpingogram) procedure (where they flush your fallopian tubes with dye to ensure there are no blockages, under x-ray guidance) and that is no picnic! I remember lying down with a nurse holding my hand while they got busy with the dye and flushed my tubes and she said, 'You're going to feel contractions now, like during labour.' I wondered whether this would be my only experience of labour-like contractions or whether it was just a preview.

While the husband/partner has little of a medical nature to endure personally throughout the investigations, he does have to provide a sperm sample for analysis. This was a pretty horrible experience for my husband because despite the letter stating they had 'facilities' for providing a sample, when we got to the hospital (a different one to the usual hospital we attended) the 'facilities' turned out to be the normal toilets... Three cubicles, all of which were clogged with shit. As this sample was small and of a low count he had to provide a repeat (public toilets aren't conducive for a quality sample then?). This time he produced the sample at home and we drove it to the hospital, arriving with merely seconds before the apparent expiry time of the sample. He didn't want to go through that experience in the public toilets again. Despite it being a rather unpleasant experience for him I was endlessly amused by it. We did complain about the 'facilities' to the consultant and she said we would have to write a letter of complaint as her comments hadn't been taken on board by the other department. We never did though, just couldn't find the right words to start a complaint letter which involved shit and wanking.

In the middle of this year of tests and long waits for appointments, my father-in-law passed away after a long and intermittent battle with cancer. This came as quite a shock to us all as he'd decided to hide the true reality of his condition from his children. After he moved to the other side I know my husband and I both felt the frustration and bitter sadness that he would never meet any of his grandchildren. I remember feeling particularly angry that my body hadn't managed to get pregnant since I'd stopped taking the pill two years ago – plenty of time to have been pregnant, given birth and been able to introduce the child to its grandfather. Alas, it was not to be, but that didn't stop it weighing heavy on our hearts. Infertility felt incredibly cruel to even rob our wider family of the experience of having a grandchild. I know this feeling of sadness stayed with us for a long time.

We were into the second half of 2010 now and it was becoming harder to be positive. The pressure had been taken off the two of us by waiting for all the test results, but the sadness was accumulating. The appointments with the consultant were few and far between and results from tests took ages, it seemed. So we were in a sort of limbo – unsure whether we really were properly infertile (or subfertile) or just taking a long time to get pregnant, so we weren't really sure how to feel. A part of us really believed that all we needed were some drugs to increase ovulation and we'd be fine. It frustrated me that we couldn't just have a prescription for Clomid – all this time waiting and waiting just seemed to be a waste.

I was spending a lot of time trawling fertility forums and looking for some information – any information – that would help us get pregnant without intervention since there was nothing forthcoming from the medical professionals. There were loads of quite crazy suggestions and most didn't have any real success rates, just anecdotal evidence. I wouldn't usually decide to join in with that sort of stuff, I might read a book someone suggested, but I wasn't going to make a drastic diet change because one person swore they got pregnant the same month. Although I might've decided to eat extra pineapple or drink extra milk if several people had said it was the way to go (of course it wasn't). I'd read a highly recommended book that sang the praises of charting your basal body temperature, so I immediately bought a thermometer and started charting my temperature every morning to see if I could note any signs of ovulation. I was charting the info on a free fertility website, but I don't think I did this for long. After a couple of months with no positive test I probably just got despondent and stopped (also I kept forgetting to take my temperature).

Someone on one of the forums mentioned that soy isoflavones (vitamins I'd never previously heard of) worked in the same way as the ovulation-boosting drug Clomid. Even if you google it today you'll find the old (and new!) forum threads with people discussing using soy isoflavones to get pregnant – or conceive multiples! I really do not think it is a good idea to just take these vitamins (and make up your own dosage or follow someone else's online), however, a woman trying to conceive and failing will try anything (within reason). If a doctor suggests it then go for it, if someone online mentions it, best to avoid or do your research first. So I decided on a particularly desperate month to give this idea a go. I have no idea what dosage or when I took the tablets but I did and there was a more obvious ovulation on my temperature chart – but this could just have been coincidence. Of course, I didn't get pregnant from that cycle and I didn't bother trying it again. I think I knew it was just a daft thing to do.

I appreciate I'm making this time in our lives sound like a psychological mess, but it's important to note that life went on as usual while this was going on behind our closed doors. We still had fun, saw friends, attended weddings, went on holiday, watched films, went to work, went on nights out, went out for meals, read books, went out for the day, all that totally normal stuff. So it wasn't as if every single day was filled with black clouds, but those clouds were always there, though often just in our peripheral vision, not right in front of our eyes. It's that shadow in a conversation, that awkward moment when someone asks you if you want kids or when you're going to have them – it's that feeling in the pit of your stomach, the knowledge that you're going to have to think of something to say to brush off the question and divert it elsewhere. So the clouds were never really absent and life was as life is, but the clouds weren't constantly in focus. No amount of positive thinking could ever make them leave.

My tests confirmed what we already knew, and in addition to PCOS, I had a large cyst next to my left ovary, which needed removing, so I was placed on a waiting list for the surgery. So, I had PCOS, more than likely was not ovulating (I wasn't during the tests anyway), I was obese and needed to lose some weight. I could see all the reasons stacked up against me being able to conceive. I couldn't quite see the same barriers on my husband's side – he was naturally slim, didn't smoke and had no health issues that seemed relevant, aside from having surgery to correct an undescended testicle when he was young. I felt it was my fault, but I didn't know what I could do other than wait for a prescription of Clomid and continue trying to lose the weight my consultant had asked me to.

All these tests took a long time to complete and despite getting the re-confirmation of PCOS reasonably quickly, the rest took much longer, for no apparent reason, and it was now over a year since we'd been referred. The consultant was happy that I had lost a little weight and began talking to me about Clomid – the drug that I had eagerly read so much about online and was hoping upon hope that she would prescribe for me. I remember sitting there thinking – finally! Finally we were going to get this drug! But then she suddenly stopped and realised that she hadn't actually reviewed my husband's lab results. Yes, she had them but hadn't actually looked at them (made me wonder if they'd had all the results quite quickly but didn't bother checking them or informing us). He wasn't with me at that appointment, as he couldn't get the time off work. The consultant scanned the results and her tone changed. He had a low sperm count. Low enough to mean that there would be no point in trying Clomid, and no point even trying IUI (intrauterine insemination – the step after that). In fact, our only option would be to go on the waiting list for IVF (in vitro fertilization – 'in vitro' means 'in glass'), because, in her words, 'He's not going to get you pregnant.'

I don't know if I felt shock or not. I know I went through the motions, filled in forms related to the treatment, got told emphatically that if I hadn't lost significant weight by the time we got to the top of the eighteen-month waiting list then I would go back on the list and wouldn't receive any treatment until the weight had been lost. I needed a BMI (body mass index) of under thirty. I would also need the surgery to remove the large cyst before any treatment started as well. I merely said okay and agreed that I would do everything I possibly could. But I went away with little idea of how on earth I would be able to do it. I'd never lost more than about two stone and I'd always ended up gaining it back. I'd lost a little weight at that point, but nothing anywhere near significant.

I drove away from the hospital and stopped near my parents' house to phone my husband. It was news I didn't want to have to impart, especially as he was at work, but I had to. He wanted to know. I think that phone call was the moment it all sunk in because I remember that telling him was incredibly difficult and I was trying not to cry – I don't think I succeeded. I felt a pit of despair opening deep inside me and blackness filling it, but I was going to see my parents and I didn't want to look upset.

Infertility can be so isolating. People are afraid of sharing because they're embarrassed that they're unable to do something that they are biologically designed to do. Admitting that your reproductive organs don't work properly is not an easy thing to do. So the majority of infertile people say nothing, get on with it, and try not to show how they feel. They smile and buy presents and congratulate their friends and family on their new babies and inside they feel like dying because they just don't understand why it isn't happening for them – why everyone else and not them? But it's only when we open up and be honest with people that we find out that it isn't just us, it's the reality for many, many people and we're not alone. But for that moment I didn't know what to say or do so I pretended everything was okay and kept driving.

From that day on, everything changed in ways I could not have predicted.

CHAPTER TWO
How the hell am I going to do this?

The night after that fateful appointment in January 2011, when I found out it was IVF or bust, I went online and googled Weight Watchers. I have no idea why I picked that particular company, but I did and I signed up online immediately. I had no knowledge of them, no preference, it was just a name that came to me. Knowing that I had close to a hundred pounds to lose made the task seem gigantic and frightening. I quite honestly didn't think I could do it. Although I had lost a little weight in the tail end of the previous year, in the past I'd never successfully lost anything for long. I'd always put the weight back on after going off plan and forgetting to get back on.

I had been weighed at my appointment with the consultant a couple of months previously and been told that I had ninety-five pounds to lose. I had managed to lose eleven pounds by that day, which the consultant had been happy about. However, I now needed to really focus and get my BMI below thirty, which meant I needed to get the remaining eighty-four pounds off as soon as I could – and I didn't have a huge amount of time to do it in. I immediately set the goal of Christmas that year, just in case the waiting list was more like twelve months rather than eighteen (wishful thinking). This was back in the days of Pro Points on Weight Watchers and much to my surprise, I found it really simple to follow. I had twenty-nine Pro Points a day, forty-nine weekly Pro Points for treats and I could eat as much fruit and vegetables as I desired. So the first week I lost four pounds. It wasn't quite the big loss I'd seen people mention on forums (I spent a lot of time lurking…) but it was a start. The second week I had a cold and one of the days I felt terribly sorry for myself so decided to eat a shit load of chocolate. I thought I was now doomed. Just another diet that I'd fail at. Great. How was I ever going to do this?

However, to my utter delight, that second week (and the second week is known for a very small loss to compensate the normally huge first week loss) I lost six pounds. I was on a high now – ten pounds in two weeks – I had never before achieved anything like that. I can only assume that God and the angels were cutting me some slack that week to encourage me to keep going. It worked. Seeing the amount I had to lose drop to seventy-four pounds so quickly was the incentive I needed to keep going. I was starting to feel like I could do this.

In the first couple of months I lost weight, but it didn't yet look all that significant. I think I went down a clothing size, so it was noticeable to me but not necessarily to everyone else. At the time I was in the middle of a teacher training course. It still baffles me as to why I ever thought that course was a good idea. I'd never, ever wanted to be a teacher and yet as I was finishing up my research degree and working in a crappy job, the idea started to appeal to me. So I'd applied and started the course the previous September, and in total honesty the first teaching term was lovely. I gelled with the teachers and the pupils and I thought I was doing the right thing.

Then Christmas came around and we had time off, then went back to university for a while and then onto the second school. In the meantime I'd found out that we were infertile and IVF treatment was our only hope, so I don't think I had anywhere near the right mindset to deal with any challenges. The second school was where it all unravelled; I unravelled. I didn't fit at all, not with the teachers, my fellow trainee teachers or the pupils. It was just a horrible experience all round. And all the while I was suffering with the secret pain of infertility and it was suffocating.

One day I got to school as normal but could not make myself leave the staff room. I went to the toilets and just started crying and couldn't stop. I panicked and quickly told the reception staff that something was wrong (there was no one else around to speak to) and I fled the school. I drove to my parents' house and I spent the day with my mum and her friend. We went out to lunch and had a look around shops in a neighbouring town. It was a blissful distraction from everything. I pretended that I had no troubles and was just on a nice day out. As soon as I'd left the school that morning I knew I could never go back without having a complete breakdown.

After this (what I refer to as) mini-breakdown I visited the doctor to discuss my mental health. She advised me to have a weekend away and take a break from the teaching course. The tutors on the course were unaccepting of this and told me that I couldn't take two weeks off, it was quit or come back straight away – that made it easier as I didn't really want to return. And I was very glad that I did make that decision because unbeknown to me, one of the teachers at the school had decided to fabricate a story about me being out blind drunk the weekend after I left the school in tears. I'd never experienced that kind of petty, childish behaviour from an adult before (but sadly I've seen it a few times since!), but as someone once said to me, some people never stop being children. It's just unfortunate this person was in a position of power teaching impressionable children.

After closing the door on that unmitigated disaster, I had to find a job quickly. I needed to find something, anything, which meant we could pay all our bills. I managed to get a job as an admin assistant quite quickly. It was meant to be a stopgap job for six months and it was a relief that I would be able to contribute towards the bills. At least we weren't going to go bankrupt during this difficult time. My weight loss continued steadily and it was really starting to make an impression on other people. I'd never lost significant weight before so it was quite shocking to friends and family.

Quite honestly I think that focusing on the weight loss programme was a distraction from everything else that was going on. Seeing the scale go down each week was my only success amongst nothing but failure. I wasn't even very happy at my MPhil (research degree) graduation in the summer. I felt that despite my viva exam being positive and being told that my thesis could easily have been developed further, it just wasn't good enough because it was one step down from a PhD. I couldn't find a way to be proud of myself for completing the degree. It makes me sad now to think that I couldn't find it in me to celebrate this massive accomplishment, but my mindset was so negative that nothing but the highest accolade or achieving my ultimate dreams would do.

Around October that year I went in to have the large cyst removed from next to my left ovary. I had keyhole surgery and I think the recovery was reasonably quick. Part of me thought that the procedure would boost my fertility but it didn't – just like the HSG procedure didn't either. My consultant was there for the procedure and she was very impressed with my weight loss – I was only a few pounds away from my target weight. I remember looking at my reflection in a toilet mirror as I stood there in my hospital gown and not recognising myself. I hoped that there wouldn't be much longer to wait before we could start our fertility treatment, but no information on timescales was forthcoming. For some reason seeing my consultant so pleased with my weight loss was the highest praise I felt I could have received at that time.

I met my weight loss target not long after the surgery and it was thrilling to have achieved something I'd never thought possible. I couldn't quite believe I'd lost ninety-five pounds. Of course, no one else around me could quite believe it either. I had gone from wearing a size twenty-two to a size twelve and it was completely unknown territory for me. My BMI was somewhere under thirty, where it needed to be. I was physically ready for the next stage and I needed to make the consultant abundantly aware of it. I went to the doctors and made them weigh me to update their records and asked them to write to the consultant to tell her that the weight was gone in the hopes that it would hurry up my treatment.

During this time of losing weight I almost felt as though it wasn't me that was really doing it. I had been obese my entire life, so how was I managing to do it with relative ease? (I say 'relative ease' because losing weight takes hard work and dedication, but I was doing it and I wasn't hating myself so that seemed easy to me.) I encountered a lot of different attitudes during this time. People were either impressed, jealous or dubious. 'How can you eat that chocolate bar if you're dieting?' 'Oh, be careful the weight doesn't go back on – you'd better not go out for a curry.'

It appeared to people that one chocolate bar or curry and whoops, that'd be me fifty pounds heavier overnight! These comments were very frustrating. I also had people messaging me asking, 'What's your secret?' Hoping that I would have some magic thing to tell them – well you go to the forest and search for the magic faerie elixir, you drink that down and then poof, the weight will fall off at a steady rate over several months... No one really liked my response of 'everything in moderation' – it was disappointing to them. Now that I'd lost the required weight, I hoped and prayed that the treatment would be just around the corner.

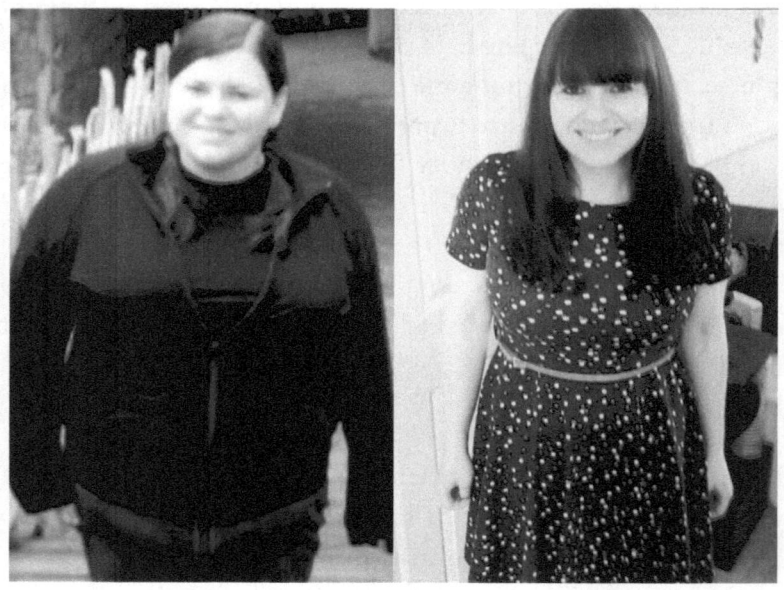

As we got into 2012, I continued to try and keep my weight down. I would gain and lose a few pounds quite often, nothing significant, and nothing that pushed my BMI over the cut-off point of thirty. Mentally, I was struggling as aside from the weight loss, I felt that I had failed at everything. I didn't feel like I could find anything to be grateful for. The weight loss hadn't seemed to help my cycle regulate or make me more fertile as I still wasn't getting pregnant naturally. Infertility had really infected my thoughts and taken me to a very dark place. I struggled to find meaning in anything.

A strange and perhaps psychologically messy part of weight loss is the odd feeling that you've turned into someone else externally, when inside you're the same person. The comments were frequent and plentiful: 'Oh you look like a different person!' 'Wow, you've lost so much weight I didn't even recognise you!' These comments are wonderful to start with, but then when coupled with seeing photographs of yourself and also struggling to recognise yourself, there's some confusion – you see, in my head I looked exactly the same as I always did. My mental image hadn't updated. I would still go to shops and look for the biggest sizes first before realising that I didn't need that size anymore.

The truth is that if you're insecure or depressed or unhappy before losing weight, the weight loss won't magically change any of that. Any existing issues will still be there. Sure, weight loss can have a multitude of health benefits, and that's wonderful, but any deep-seated issues present before will still need addressing after. Losing weight won't sort anyone's life out for them. I know this for certain. I've heard so many people comment that if they could just lose ten, twenty or fifty pounds, then their life would be fantastic, but you don't lose your issues along with the weight, those issues remain with you regardless. I'm not saying I wasn't pleased with my achievement, because I was, I was delighted that I'd managed to achieve something I'd never thought possible, but even after I'd lost the weight, I was still looking for a distraction from the dark clouds.

The distraction I needed arrived in the form of exercise. In April that year a friend of mine ran the London Marathon, something which I was utterly in awe of. His achievement really made me want to join in and start running myself. Yes, I'd lost all that weight but I had done it entirely through diet, no exercise at all, which some people may find difficult to believe. But just focusing on my diet was enough for me at that time. Adding exercise as well might have been too overwhelming.

But I was ready now, so I started with Jillian Michaels' at home workout DVDs, as recommended by a friend. I started with the very popular 30 Day Shred DVD and just went for it. I wanted to start running, but at the time I was simply too self-conscious to run outside, so I stuck to the DVDs. Looking back, it seems a little daft that I was too self-conscious to run outside after losing all that weight, but, as I said before, my mental image of myself hadn't yet updated and I felt far more comfortable working out at home, away from the gaze of strangers. I also thought that building up a good base of fitness would help me when I did start running. I didn't want to get out there, only be able to run for thirty seconds then give up and go home.

Over the next few months I worked out six days a week, as well as continuing to monitor my diet, and I lost more weight. My total weight loss at that point was a hundred and three pounds. I found that through exercise I had really found a wonderful way of helping myself. It improved my mental health, and really aided my physical fitness and wellbeing. I relished the endorphins that were released with each workout and the strong feeling of accomplishment. I looked forward to seeing improvements in my fitness levels week after week, as it felt like consistent success. It was a very positive influence in my life. Now I was wearing clothes between size eight, ten and twelve, shop dependent, and I was quite pleased with myself – this, coupled with my new found love of exercise, was the only thing that I managed to feel pleased about. Infertility and all the connected issues still weighed heavily. Despite all the distractions, I still kept waiting for a letter or phone call to tell us that our treatment was due to begin. As we had now exceeded the eighteen-month wait, I started to think it was never going to happen.

Chapter Three
Positivity, where are you?

There was a full year between reaching the required weight goal and starting the first IVF cycle. Aside from adding exercise into my days, going to work and editing the odd book, I didn't really have anything else to do other than dwell. I found my spare time was mostly dominated by negative thoughts. I came to the realisation that I had always been a pessimist. My attitude all along had been: have low expectations, you can't be disappointed then. This now sounds awful to me, but it was completely normal at the time and had been for as long as I could remember. Despite growing up in a religious household (my stepfather was a minister) I had never been overly religious myself. I'd spent a significant portion of my childhood in various churches, but at this time I only went to church occasionally. In truth, I'd always struggled with it, I felt half atheist and half Christian.

After I had lost the weight and was physically ready for treatment but still waiting, something inside me wanted to find a more positive way of living, even if it was just a better way to order my thoughts. I was aware that a close friend of mine was spiritual (she's an author of spiritual fiction) so I asked for her help. I wasn't comfortable seeking help in any other way at that point, religious or not. I trusted her completely so I knew she would understand. She introduced me to an entirely different way of thinking and to new concepts and ideas about faith and spirituality and our own personal relationships with God or the universe. She sent me a few books to read and I slowly began reading and learning more and more about life as a more spiritual and positive person.

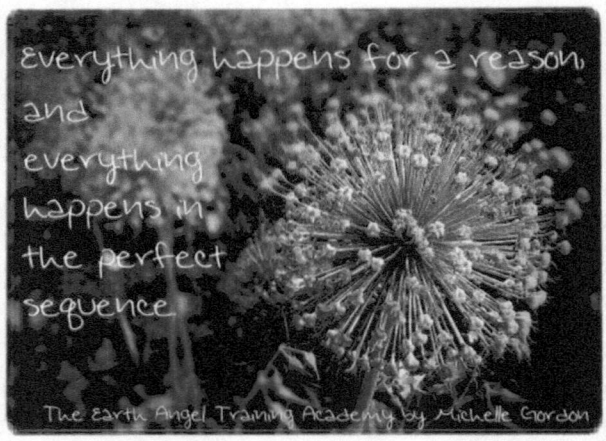

I began to repeat positive affirmations to myself, which was very calming and evoked a feeling of safety. I appreciate this isn't everyone's cup of tea, but for me it just felt right. Of course, at first I struggled with certain aspects. If I decided to say a positive affirmation such as 'I am safe' my brain would go into overdrive with questions – am I safe though? How do I know I'm safe? Am I lying to myself? Exhausting. But slowly these positive affirmations became calming and they helped ground me to the present moment. 'I am currently safe in my location therefore I am safe.' Positive affirmations can be used to help us focus on things that we want as well, so for example, if I was starting to feel panic arising, I could tell myself 'I am calm' or 'I am healthy' and focus on my breathing to keep the anxiety under control.

Another helpful tool was meditation, which is something I didn't do all that regularly, but I always felt better if I'd done it. I preferred guided meditation as otherwise my mind wandered a bit too much. Even with the guided meditations, there was always a bit of mind wandering at the start but after a while it calmed down. On a particularly low or anxious day, setting aside time to meditate was very helpful. Even if I ended up falling asleep, I hoped my mind still took in the positivity from the guidance in the meditation, and if it wasn't guided then at least I had relaxed myself and calmed down. I generally found these meditations on YouTube, but you can download apps for your phone as well.

I found that gratitude was incredibly important. It sounds very simple, but the mere act of counting your blessings and finding things to be thankful for every day really works wonders. They can be as big or as small as you like – from being grateful that you've found your life partner to being thankful that you had a slice of cake earlier. What you're doing is getting yourself to focus on the good in your life and not allowing yourself to dwell on the bad. If you make a list or just think about what you are grateful for today then you are bringing more good to yourself, as you will see the good more often.

If we focus on the bad and negative things we will see more of the same, so if the option is there to notice more good and that helps you feel happier, why not do it? We all have so much to be grateful for, even when we struggle to see it. If we have a home to live in, electricity, running water, food to eat, clothes to wear, etc., we have so much to be thankful for. Negativity attracts negativity; positivity attracts positivity.

I found that focusing on gratitude helped with consciously trying to improve my thoughts and then eventually helped with replacing negative thoughts with positive ones. I don't think we truly realise how negative our thoughts and speech can be, so being as mindful as possible about what we are thinking and saying means we can correct ourselves and make an effort to speak more positively. For example, if I was nervous about a job interview, instead of doing what I'd usually do and tell myself that I wouldn't get the job and think about all the awful things that could happen, I would imagine a positive experience and outcome, and tell myself that I was suitable, qualified and worthy of the job. If I didn't end up getting the job, that would mean there was something better for me out there and I wasn't meant to get that particular job. This would then lead to me being calmer and more confident and talkative in the interview rather than being a bag of nerves, assuming the worst before I'd even arrived.

I've had issues with focusing on failure, and I've lost count of how many times I've counted my failures again and again. So one way I've tried to combat this is through gratitude or focusing on the good instead. Every time I might've got bogged down thinking about all the ways in which I've failed, I've switched the focus straight away thought about all the successes, big or small, and then thought about those again and again. I turned negative thoughts into positive ideas and I am thankful for all the good I've experienced in my life.

Prayer can be powerful. I know not everyone thinks it's worth their time, as it has very religious connotations, but praying instead of worrying helps release tension and fear. 'Give it to God' is a well-known saying and that's pretty much what prayer is. It doesn't matter who you are praying to – God, the angels, the universe, yourself – what matters is that you're taking your fears, your worries and instead of dwelling on them over and over and living in those worries, you're sending them away through prayer. You're asking for help, asking for guidance, and it's a very peaceful process not unlike meditation. If asking for guidance, you'll be surprised where the answer or help then comes from, but you'll notice it and you'll see the connection.

One of the most difficult (in my experience) parts of living a more positive (and spiritual) life is accepting negative experiences as learning opportunities. At this point in our infertility journey I really wasn't in a place to accept any of the difficult experiences and learn from them, as I had no distance to be able to see them for what they were. This was something that would come to me in time (after more difficult experiences), but I was starting to be able to connect the dots between why things happened. Everything happens for a reason, after all. I'd started remembering things from the past and was making an effort to accept that those things happened and acknowledge what I learnt from them. I was trying to see the bigger picture. But it was still too early for me to understand and learn from our situation at the time.

Something that is deeply connected to seeing the bigger picture is accepting and releasing the past and forgiving yourself and others, a tall order, but one that brings significant peace. Quite often we'll store hate, resentment and shame within ourselves and carry it around with us. It weighs heavy. Again, I cannot say that at this point, or at any point since, that I have been completely successful in releasing and forgiving. But just making an effort to try and accept that someone who may have hurt you did so for reasons other than you can see from your perspective, and then forgiving and releasing them, really does take some of that weight away, leaving a lighter, easier energy behind.

There is no need to condone anyone's behaviour or suddenly decide that what happened was okay, but forgiving them and releasing what you've been holding onto is a good way of shedding negativity from your life. This includes forgiving yourself. In fact, if you only manage to forgive one person it needs to be yourself. I have struggled with self-forgiveness a lot. I have dwelled and re-lived things from my life and hated myself for how things were. Understanding that everything that happened needed to happen and acknowledging that I have no reason not to forgive myself has brought great peace. We are all human, subject to error, and forgiveness is something we all deserve. It is freeing.

Another activity which can be very helpful is creating a vision board or diary. I was quite sceptical of doing this at first, but making the effort to print or collect and stick photos of what you'd like in your life to a board, or in a book, or writing down what you would like to happen in a diary (in positive present tense) is a great way to focus. This board can be used for motivation or you can even just put it away and know that you've sent your intention out into the universe. I favour writing the bigger things down and having pictures of the smaller things on a board. Examples that I have personally written are: 'A baby will come to us at the right time.' 'I can run the London Marathon.' 'I have relocated to a new house.' Equally, photos that depict the same meaning would be great, as long as you know the intention and meaning behind the image, it will have the same impact.

You can also just make it really simple, and make a list of things that make you feel better and then on a difficult day revisit it. Read your favourite book, watch your favourite film, go away for the weekend, bake a cake (but try not to eat it all by yourself in one go), or indulge yourself in something you like doing: crafting, walking, etc. Find ways and reasons to make the day great. And never lose your sense of humour. There are always comedic moments, even in the darkest of times, believe me.

I can't pretend that I was always super positive from this point onwards, but it gave me something to think about, do and focus on during bad times, especially with the dark clouds circling. Making the decision to be positive really helped me change my attitude to my life at that point. Simply thinking positive doesn't necessarily solve anything, but it might help you feel a bit better, especially if it's alongside other steps towards healing. I started to believe that I could do what I wanted, that I could have a baby, that I could be happy. It built me up to feel good about our approaching IVF treatment and helped me gain a better mindset.

Chapter Four
When reproduction needs assistance

One thing that struck me quite significantly about assisted reproduction, IVF in particular, is how little people seemed to know or understand about it. Because we had made the decision relatively early on to be open about our impending treatment (especially since people kept asking me why I had decided to lose weight), we would get the oddest comments in return. I had people assume that IVF happened in one day – you'd go in in the morning and leave in the afternoon pregnant. As if it was that easy. People seemed to generally believe that IVF equalled a baby. With all those scientists and test tubes and stuff there was no chance of it not producing a baby, surely? There were also some ill-informed comments like: 'Aren't all children born from IVF sterile? Obese? Diabetic? Generally ill?' Um, what? And many other questions, from the general to the daft, such as how do they get the egg from you? How do they put the embryo back? Does it really grow in a test tube? Can you choose if it's a boy or a girl? Why do they freeze stuff sometimes? Do they do research on the embryos? How developed is it before they put it in your womb? Will you have to stay lying down for days after the embryo transfer to stop it falling out? And, of course, there were the people who felt that any fertility treatment was messing with nature and shouldn't be allowed. But that argument doesn't hold water. Infertility is defined as a disease by the World Health Organisation and should be treated like any other. If all other diseases are worthy of treatment, why should infertility be any different?

We had taken the time to educate ourselves on the procedure and the failure and success rates, and had a hopeful but realistic viewpoint about the whole thing. I was more than happy to believe it would work first time. After all, I'd lost the weight specifically for this treatment, so that we could finally be pregnant with our first child. Surely it was now our time? We had good odds on our side. We were young and healthy, our sperm and eggs just needed a little assistance.

Something that I found difficult to deal with were the inappropriate comments we received from people who were close to us or people we knew who'd had no issues with fertility themselves. 'You know, I wouldn't have gone through this – I wouldn't have done IVF if I couldn't have kids.' Right... what do you want me to take away from that? Either you don't think we should have this treatment for whatever reason, or you don't think having your own children is very important or worth it. Or maybe you're belittling the blight that infertility places over a person's life. Or perhaps you just do not understand. I always chose to believe that they just didn't understand because it made the comments easier to deal with.

I'd also have people bring up storylines or characters from films or TV shows who couldn't have children. Right... what do you want me to say to that? 'I saw this film and there was a woman who couldn't have children so they never had any.' Uh, right, that's interesting. 'I read about this famous woman who had IVF four times and still didn't get pregnant, how is that possible?' Because IVF isn't a magic wand. 'You'll be too old for this treatment by the time you reach the end of this waiting list!' Since I'm in my twenties, I don't think that's something I need to worry about, thanks. Sometimes comments were hurtful, though. And just because you've been open with them about it all, it doesn't mean you want to be used as an example and have the topic brought up at any moment that suits them either.

Then there are the people who think they are being nice and helpful and encouraging by telling you brand new information, when all they are really doing is repeating the same old unhelpful stuff everyone else does. Relax and it'll happen, stop trying and it'll happen, people fall pregnant on the waiting list for treatment, you know. Plenty of babies need adoption, why don't you adopt? Have you tried monitoring your ovulation with ovulation tests? Go on holiday and you'll fall pregnant... No one gets to the point of needing IVF without trying everything possible to conceive naturally, it comes across as insulting to our intelligence that people think otherwise. No one undertakes difficult treatment without it being their last resort. No medical professional would allow you to undertake the treatment unless it was your last resort.

I do understand why people decide to keep this process to themselves, because it really is an immensely personal thing to go through. As open as I was about it all, there were days when I didn't want to talk about it and then people struggled to see how it was okay to discuss it yesterday, but not today. Personally, I just felt that it was too big a thing to go through to keep entirely to ourselves; I wanted to be able to talk about it. I felt it was important to do so because infertility is quite often a taboo subject and people are afraid to discuss it because they are embarrassed or ashamed. Wanting something and then being unable to have it is difficult, regardless of what it is. But when it's the inability to have children, this really strikes you at your core. We are biologically designed to reproduce, it should be as easy and natural as any of our other functions, so when you can't achieve this one thing that seemingly everyone else finds so easy to achieve, it really does shake up everything you know and believe in. It leaves an undeniable feeling of failure surrounding you.

And then someone would say, 'Oh I only had to look at him and we'd be pregnant,' or 'He only had to brush past me on the stairs and I'd be pregnant again,' and it would cement all the irrational thoughts about failure into your mind as fact. It makes you think that yes, it is easy for everyone else and you must be defective in some way. Infertility really buries its way into your brain and taunts you... every pregnant woman you see, every father with kids walking down the street, every pregnancy or birth announcement, it digs away at your wellbeing, making you feel as though you are less of a person. Of course, the rational side of you may try and step in and tell you you're just being silly – there's nothing wrong with you, having a baby doesn't make you a better person, not having a baby doesn't make you a failure, a person's worth isn't measured by their reproductive organs – but when you're there, in the middle of the darkness, no one can tell you any differently.

In the autumn of 2012, we finally received a letter in the post. We would begin our IVF treatment when my next menstrual cycle started, so we needed to go to in to have an initial consultation to organise the treatment plan. I was nervously excited. Excited because we were finally getting our treatment and nervous because I had to undertake all of the injections and procedures. I was also overwhelmed because this treatment was a lot to take on board.

After our first consultation, we had all the information we needed. We would be having ICSI (intra-cytoplasmic sperm injection), which is IVF, but instead of the sperm and the egg being left to their own devices for fertilisation in a dish, a single sperm would be injected into the egg to give the process a further helping hand. This procedure is generally used for those with a low sperm count or with other issues with sperm.

The treatment would start by down-regulating, which would consist of daily injections of Buserelin (in the morning, in my case) to stop any natural cycle from happening. After about two weeks of these morning injections, the follicle stimulating hormone injection of Menopur would start in the early evening (in my case). These would continue for around two weeks to stimulate the ovaries to release eggs. Ultrasounds would take place throughout the process to monitor the progress. When a scan would confirm enough follicles were present and of a suitable size, the egg collection would be booked and there would be a third, one time only, injection of hCG (Human Chorionic Gonadotrophin) about thirty-six hours prior to mature the eggs quickly ready for collection.

During the egg collection I would be sedated or given a light general anaesthetic and a long needle would be sent up through the vagina and into each ovary to take the eggs away. This would be done under ultrasound for guidance. Just before I'd have this retrieval, my husband would provide a sperm sample. After recovery, we'd be sent home and the embryologists would then get to work assisting the egg and sperm to fertilise in the lab. The successfully fertilised eggs would then grow in the lab for a few days before being transferred back to my uterus. I would then be given hormonal medication (usually a pessary) to get the womb lining ready to receive one or two embryos at transfer. This medication is continued until a pregnancy test is taken (if negative the medication is stopped, if positive it is continued for a while into pregnancy).

During the transfer the embryos would be sent into the womb using a catheter, sometimes under ultrasound guidance, sometimes not. If not, the equipment is checked after the procedure to ensure no embryos are still present. Two weeks later a pregnancy test (standard shop-bought test) would be taken to find out if the treatment has been successful.

Even though I knew all this, having read widely on the topic, hearing it explained and realising that it was actually happening to us was quite surreal. I was given medication to force my period to start (Norethisterone) because with PCOS I could never guarantee when it would start, and we began our first cycle in October. For this cycle, my medication was delivered to the house. I laid it all out to look at everything before storing it (some of it needed refrigerating). The sheer number of needles and syringes and bottles was frightening. Would it really take all of this to help us get pregnant? After panicking a little, I tried to change my mindset – each medication, each injection would be taking us closer to having a baby, so I did my best to feel thankful for each dose. My husband was to do my injections, as he'd been trained by the nurse. I thought this was a good idea because it involved him more in the process – a process which is undeniably heavily centred on the female.

After my treatment cycle began and the down-regulation started, it felt like we were on our way. We were getting used to the morning injections, despite several unnecessary panics about air bubbles on my part, and I was starting to feel the side effects of having my natural cycle repressed – it's pretty much like a temporary menopause. I'm not sure if it's common to have side effects or whether you just feel a bit more on edge mood-wise,

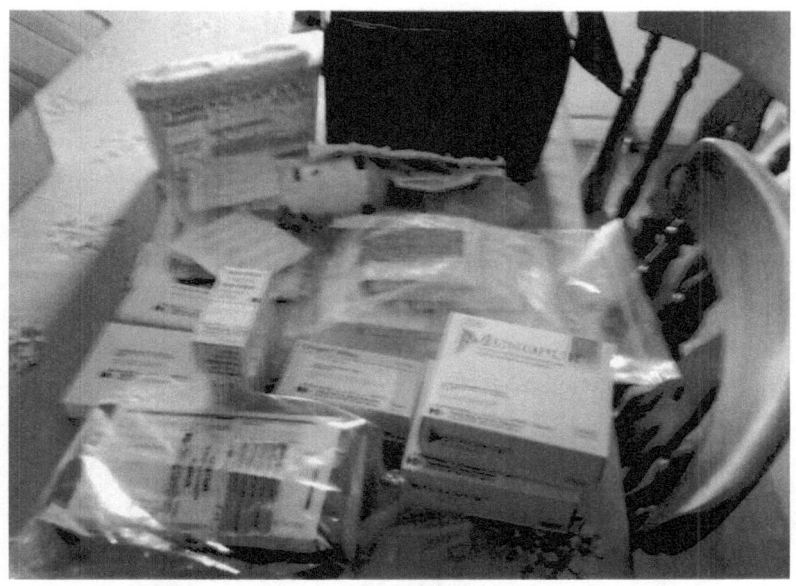

The IVF drugs

but I do remember feeling moody and down quite a lot. My husband was doing well with the injections, but on one or two occasions I had to do them myself, including one time in the car due to an early clinic appointment. I remember completely freaking out and couldn't make myself do it. I was crying in the car and hoping no one could see me. It took me several attempts to complete the injection successfully and I took a while afterwards to calm down. I soon got over this experience, however. I think it was more the emotions of the entire experience that affected me rather than the individual injection itself.

However, despite the few personal panics, all was progressing well and an ultrasound scan showed that the down-regulating injections had done what they were meant to do. So we then started the second daily injection, the follicle stimulating hormone injections (Menopur). This one was a bit trickier, maybe not for everyone but it was for us. This medication needed to be mixed. There was a bottle of powder and a glass vial of pure water. You snapped off the top of the glass bottle and tipped the water into the other bottle to mix with the powder. I'm not exactly sure why we had such trouble with this, but we were often accidentally smashing the glass and having to use another one instead. I think nerves probably contributed to that. Starting the second injections meant that I started to feel a bit better because these injections were to build up, not to shut down like the other ones, and because it meant we were progressing with the treatment cycle and getting closer to our goal.

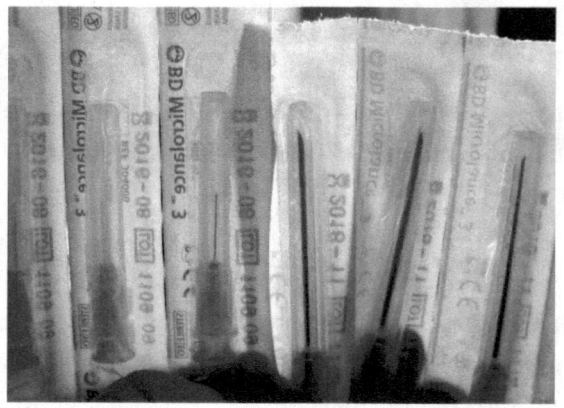

The injecting needles and mixing needles. At first I panicked and thought the mixing needles were for injecting!

There were other side effects during this part: sore breasts, abdominal discomfort, and I continued to be prone to mood swings. Psychologically, it was an unusual and daunting experience. Sometimes I felt like a bit of a crazy woman.

I remember getting a lot of phone calls from the clinic during the cycle. Aside from arranging dates and times for procedures and maybe getting updates on blood results or scans, I can't think what these must have been about. At this point I was primarily only working mornings and due to having limited phone signal at our house I always felt more comfortable staying in town in case someone should ring. My husband would finish after five, the usual time, so I would wander around town and sit in Starbucks in case I should need to answer my phone. I think largely this was just an excuse not to go home. If I went home then I would be stagnant, but staying in town and walking around or watching the world go by, or even driving around, meant I was moving and I could distract myself.

It also seemed to give me the opportunity to use my imagination a little more. I would walk around shops and imagine all the things I would need to buy once the baby was born. I would sit and drink a coffee, eat a cinnamon swirl and daydream about pushing a double buggy around the shops. I would sometimes look for signs that everything was going to be okay. I suppose I was creating a little dream world for myself in the hours between myself finishing work and my husband finishing work, and there was something comforting about it. Back at home I'd see all the medication, I'd be getting ready for the evening injection and some of the fear might creep back in. I was trying so hard to remain positive.

Sometimes, someone might suggest to me that the treatment would be unsuccessful, probably in an attempt to keep me grounded in case it didn't work, and to stop the disappointment from seeming so gigantic, but I hated that. I always said that I couldn't go through with the treatment unless I felt it was going to work. Surely starting such invasive and difficult treatment with a negative mindset could only hurt our chances and make everything feel so much harder?

At one of the check-up ultrasounds it was noted that my follicle growth wasn't as great as it should be, so my dose of Menopur was doubled from then on. I had been prescribed a low dose initially due to my age (I was in my late twenties at the time). This increased dose did its job and soon enough they were happy with the follicle number and growth. It was time to book the egg collection and move into the final stage. Some women at this stage might unfortunately experience OHSS (ovarian hyperstimulation syndrome), which means the ovaries have gone into overdrive and it can be very serious, even life threatening. But I wasn't in danger of experiencing this, luckily.

At this point, we really felt like our dream of having our own child was within our reach. It was as though everything had been building up to this. All the heartache, the weight loss, the waiting, it was all leading up to the positive pregnancy test I was sure we were going to see soon. I felt confident that it was going to work. I repeated positive affirmations to myself when I felt my faith wavering and I kept believing.

Thirty-six hours before my egg collection, I remember doing the last injection, the hCG injection, to prepare the eggs ready for retrieval. I was so scared but yet grateful for the experience, it was a real mix of emotions. I remember my husband injecting that final needle into my stomach, joining the pattern of bruises from all the previous injections, and knowing that we had now done all that we could do.

Due to some issues at our fertility clinic (which was just being developed) we had to travel to a clinic across the border in England for our egg collection and transfer. We left our house very early that morning to make the long journey. It wasn't quite light yet and all the street lights were still illuminated. I remember sitting in the car, listening to the radio and looking out the window – the street lights were making little rainbows reflect on the car windows. I took this as a good sign and felt uplifted. Our treatment was taking place at a private clinic and everyone seemed nice and welcoming. I was going to have a light general anaesthetic for my egg collection, so all I remember was climbing on to the bed in the theatre, the anaesthetic being administered, and then waking back up on the ward a while later with my husband by my side. I was blissfully unaware of the procedure that had taken place. I remember drinking hot chocolate, and eating sandwiches, yogurt and fruit, which the clinic had provided during recovery.

We had to stay there for a few hours before we could head home. The embryologist came to see us not long before I was discharged to tell us that they had managed to retrieve ten eggs. I remember feeling a tad disappointed, after all, I'd read about women having far more eggs collected than that. I was pensive about this during the drive home, but I was also immensely thankful that they had ten eggs (and a few million sperm from my husband) to work with. After all, we only needed one good quality embryo for a two-day transfer or blastocyst for a five-day transfer. I went home to rest and waited for the phone call from the embryologist the next day. I remember telling friends and family about the experience and they were all hopeful, it seemed that everyone wanted this to work for us.

The next day, the embryologist rang and she had good news for us. Two eggs had fertilised and they wanted to do a two-day embryo transfer, putting both fertilised eggs into my uterus. This was it, we were going to have twins. It was amazing. I don't remember what happened to the other eight eggs. I know nothing was frozen, so perhaps they weren't of a suitable quality or they suffered failed fertilisation, I'm not sure. I was now on a high again, it really was thrilling. I couldn't wait to share the news with my husband. We were both definitely excited when we arrived back at the clinic for our embryo transfer. We sat in the ward and waited to be called in. I was wearing a dressing gown and slippers I had brought from home.

When we were called into theatre I took a moment to look around at how funny it seemed, futuristic almost. I had to sit in this huge chair, which then raised up in the air and then tipped backwards, so that my pelvis was up higher than my head and my legs were in some sort of stirrups apart – so dignified. I asked if I should take my slippers off, but she said no because it was cold in that room. It was at this moment I smelled that unmistakable smell of cat urine and realised that one of the cats must have had an accident that morning and I must have walked through it unknowingly, probably too distracted by the forthcoming procedure. Of course, then all I could think about was this poor technician smelling my cat's piss. It was a bit of comic relief at a very surreal moment. I was up in the air, in this bizarre chair surrounded by futuristic-looking medical equipment and feeling quite vulnerable. They showed us photos of the developing embryos on a screen and then someone else brought them in with the catheter. The woman fed the tubes into my vagina and into the womb and flushed the embryos out of the tubes. The catheter was then sent for examination to make sure the embryos weren't still in there. All clear. The embryos were in my womb. We had done it. I remember mentally wishing the embryos love and prayed that they would implant and grow successfully.

I went home PUPO (pregnant until proven otherwise) and settled in for the two-week wait. When anyone is trying to conceive the two-week wait between ovulation and testing becomes a time of impatience, obsession and hope, but the IVF two-week wait was extreme. The only medication to continue at this point were the progesterone pessaries, so I was inserting those daily to support the potential pregnancy. My faith that IVF had worked was very great. I knew I was pregnant. I just knew it. Each day that went by brought more nerves and more anticipation for finally seeing a positive pregnancy test, a seemingly mythical thing I'd never seen before.

I had worked out the babies' due date, I had googled everything about what to do and what not to do when pregnant. I had googled everything I could about twin pregnancies and looking after twin babies. I had refreshed my mind on what to expect in the first few weeks of pregnancy, checked when I should expect morning sickness, when I should get my first signs of a bump – sooner rather than later since there were two babies. I was all set for this next adventure.

One day when out shopping I had stopped for a (decaf) coffee break and I had panicked after ordering an eggnog latte in Starbucks without realising it might have contained raw eggs and then was too worried to drink it. I was living the role of the expectant mother, because I knew I was expecting. The fleeting thoughts about it not working were no match for how I felt inside. I wanted to go and buy a couple of baby things, just to get started, but after talking with my husband we decided to wait until we had the positive test. It would be something to look forward to. I had mentally planned the nursery and looked online for all the things we would need. We'd picked out two names, one for a girl, one for a boy. We were ready.

At some point during the two-week wait I went shopping with a close friend, and I bought a digital test and a normal test ready to use. She had listened to me go on and on about infertility and IVF over the weeks and months and years and had been a never-ending support for me. She really believed that the treatment was going to be successful as well. It was finally happening and these tests were going to prove it. I'd had no bleeding at all and I felt okay.

When the day arrived I woke up very early in the morning naturally, as you do when you're nervous about something happening later in the day. My husband was still asleep. I took the two tests to the bathroom, which was two floors down from our bedroom, and did both of them. Trembling, I waited for the results to show up. I was most excited about the digital test. I couldn't wait to see the word 'pregnant' alongside the weeks. Something about seeing the actual word would make it extra special and very real. I couldn't take my eyes off the test. I wasn't aware of anything else around me – the cats meowing for their breakfast, the coldness of the floor under my bare feet, the rain hammering against the window – it was just me and that test in that moment.

The digital test flashed up 'not pregnant'.

I stared at the test in quiet disbelief. I think I shook it to see if that might make the result change. I didn't know how to process the two words looking up at me, clear as day. What? Not pregnant? How was this possible? Surely this had to be wrong? My period hadn't arrived. I felt as if I was pregnant. It had to be wrong! I had a quick look at the other test, but couldn't see an obvious second line, so just set it aside. I didn't know what to do. I don't think I cried at that point. I felt numb. How could I go through all that just to not be pregnant at the end of it? I left the bathroom and took the tests with me into the kitchen. I didn't know what I should do at that point. I knew I had to go back to bed to wake my husband and inform him of the result, but I didn't want to. I wanted to sit downstairs, watch the rain out of the window and pretend that I hadn't yet taken the tests. I climbed the stairs slowly. I'd left the tests in the kitchen. I didn't think showing him negative tests would make it any better. I got back into bed and told him. I don't think he said anything either. We didn't know how to deal with a negative result. I cried for a while but still didn't really say anything.

Neither of us said much and we weren't going to tell anyone else the result immediately. So we managed to get up to face the day as usual. I decided to go back to the kitchen to retrieve the tests and throw them away. There was no use keeping them. I had a glance at the digital test, just in case the result had magically changed. It hadn't, so I threw it into the bin. I then took a second look at the normal, non-digital test, which I had merely glanced at before – hang on… there was a very faint pink line. I felt the hope build up and all the possibilities came alive in my mind again. I yelled for my husband to come over and showed him the test. Surely he could see this faint line as well? He could, but coupled with the definitively negative digital test, he was wary about getting our hopes up. But the hope was still there and we were both clinging onto it now. This hope was fast becoming a life raft to stop us from sinking. We decided that I would test again the next morning, so we went out and bought a couple more of the same non-digital test for the next morning and the days after. Having to wait until the next morning to test again was a huge challenge. I just wanted to know for sure that we were pregnant, not have this 'are we, are we not?' confusion.

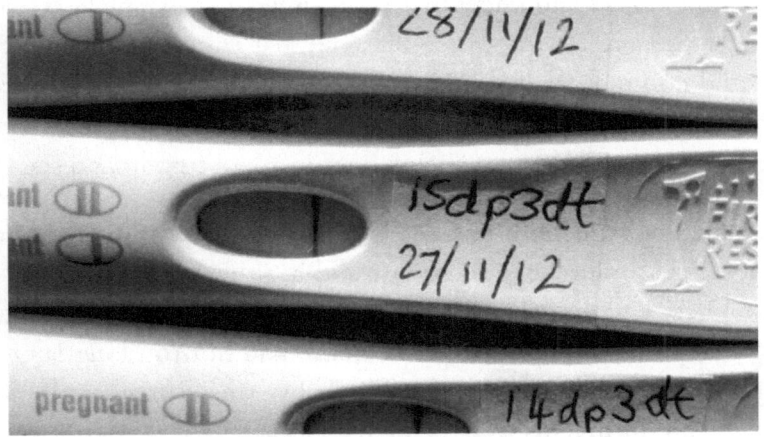

The next morning, the second line was there and it was darker. Our hope swelled. The next morning it was darker again. The morning after it was even more so. We were pregnant after all. I avoided any more digital tests because I was now afraid of what words they might display. I told everyone the truth of the situation. That the tests had been a bit confusing and that I was going to get the clinic to confirm the result for peace of mind, but also that we were pregnant. I was up and down with emotion. That first digital test had cast doubt over everything, even over these positive tests we were now seeing. I just wanted to get to the first scan so that we could see the tiny babies in there growing healthily and strongly.

However, the morning I was due to go to the hospital, the at home test (I was testing daily) had suddenly become lighter again. The fear set in. I told myself that a line was a line but something inside told me that something wasn't right. I was filled with anguish all the way to the clinic. I provided a urine sample and they sent it off to test. When the nurse came back I couldn't read her face but it was clear that she wasn't smiling. The test was positive, but it wasn't a strong positive. She said the important thing was that it was positive and I needed to continue to act and know that I was pregnant, but she also told me to prepare for the worst. She said that either the pregnancy would continue or it wouldn't and only time would tell. There was little the urine tests could show us at this point, and they didn't do blood tests routinely, so we just had to wait and see.

I remember driving home and begging my body to hold on to the babies and to keep them safe and healthy. I didn't know if I could cope with it all going wrong after it taking so long to get to this point. But life had other plans, and not too long later I started bleeding heavily, and at merely five weeks pregnant it was all over. Our dreams were being bled away.

CHAPTER FIVE
Run for your life

It took weeks and weeks to stop bleeding after the early miscarriage. I found it hard to feel positive about anything. I had so believed that it would work and that we would have twin babies, but that was now over. I swung between heartbreak and acting braver than I felt. I wasn't completely devoid of hope, however, as I knew we could have another IVF treatment cycle at some point. A few weeks after the miscarriage we had an appointment with the consultant to discuss what happened in the first cycle. As nothing really went wrong with the cycle (the only issue had been the need to increase the dose of Menopur), it was stated that the early miscarriage was just one of those unfortunate things and there wasn't anything we could have done about it. I was eager to get the second cycle underway as soon as possible, but the consultant told us we had to wait until well into the new year. We went away from this meeting disappointed. More waiting. I was geared up to continue immediately. I wanted to do the treatment straight away so that I could be pregnant again.

We were both struggling to come to terms with what had

happened and found Christmas and all the festivities very difficult to deal with. I remember standing and watching a Christmas parade in the town where my parents now lived. I saw families standing on the pavement watching the parade, all bundled up in hats and scarves, holding their babies close to their chests in baby carriers, and I said to myself in my head: 'This time next year I will stand here and watch this parade with my own baby.' I needed that bit of hope to help me through the Christmas period. I needed something to help dilute the pain of the miscarriage. I also needed something to take my mind off everything; I needed a focus. I'd put on some weight during the treatment, which is a common thing to occur, so I was conscious that I wanted to get back to the necessary BMI in case we should be contacted sooner rather than later to start our second cycle. I was only a few pounds over where I needed to be, but with the indulgence of Christmas, including extra comfort eating and drinking to try and make myself feel better, I needed to be mindful.

No one really knew what to say to us at this point, they were astounded that IVF hadn't worked. Surely IVF always works, doesn't it? It guarantees you a baby, right? No. No it doesn't. It also doesn't place you in a protective bubble to shield you and the pregnancy from any potential issues. An IVF pregnancy is as vulnerable or as strong as any other pregnancy. I was as honest as I could be with people, but more than anything I just wanted to be alone. I leaned on any method of positive thinking I could find at this point to try and help me cope with the heartbreak of losing the babies. I had known they were there from two day old embryos, so even though it was an early miscarriage, I felt I'd known them longer than I would have if it had been a natural pregnancy.

Since I had experienced so many benefits from exercising in between the weight loss and the IVF treatment, I decided to undertake a twelve-week training programme to give me something to work towards and focus on. I started Jillian Michaels' Body Revolution in early January 2013, after my husband's birthday, and I really went for it. I was doubling the workouts (doubling wasn't necessary but it was something I just wanted to do) and was getting an hour done before work. The focus really saved me at that time. I needed it. Working out first thing in the morning (even though it meant getting up very early) would put me in a good mood to face the day. I ate healthily as well and the weight came off quickly. By the end of the twelve weeks I had lost the weight I'd gained and more. I was now a hundred and ten pounds less than my previous weight back at the start. I felt really fit as well, and I felt good about my body, something which I had lost after the miscarriage – I had been angry with my body, furious that even with all that treatment it still couldn't manage to achieve a successful pregnancy. But now I was feeling comfortable and had worked hard to update how I mentally saw myself. I finally felt like I could go outside and start running.

To give myself a push out the door, I signed up for a 10k event, due to take place in only five weeks' time. People thought I was crazy, but it felt like a target was needed to motivate me. I remember my first run very clearly. I got up at the crack of dawn and snuck out, hoping that I wouldn't see anyone. I had no route in mind, I just went out and gave it a go. I was painfully slow and stopped for walking breaks (there were lots of hills) but I still managed over three miles. I got that runner's high that I'd heard people mention and I immediately loved it. I got home and felt uplifted which was a welcome feeling.

I was still struggling psychologically with the trauma of the loss and the mentally difficult IVF process as a whole, and my husband was feeling the same. Neither of us knew how to deal with it and we both blamed ourselves for our infertility. I felt like even more of a failure now than I had done when we embarked upon the treatment. I felt utterly useless and very low. Every time there would be a pregnancy announcement or a scan photo on Facebook I would cry. I would feel wretched for being unable to feel happy for whoever it was. I just felt like the sky was dark but I couldn't see a star anywhere.

This is where running became a mind clearing experience for me. I would go out early in the morning, run whatever distance I needed to for my training plan and I would feel a psychological boost. It was very similar to how I felt working out to the fitness DVDs, but somehow more so. I think getting outside and watching the miles go by had a wonderful way of allowing my mind to work through things. I always felt better afterwards. And though I was not particularly fast, I could cover the miles well. At the beginning of the year I had also made the decision to write a blog about my infertility and fitness experiences. This also became a good outlet for me to talk and work through issues. I'd received messages from people suffering with infertility who were happy to find someone willing to talk about it so openly and how they found my positive approach helpful and encouraging, which made it all worthwhile.

When the day of the 10k arrived I was nervous. It was the Race for Life 10k in Cardiff. I'd run almost six miles in training but I think there's always extra pressure when it's an official event. I had 6.2 miles to run and I was doubting whether I could do it. It was raining. My husband was ill so couldn't come to support me. My mum and sister were going to try and turn up at the end so that we could all go out for lunch, so I held onto the hope that I would see them. I got to the start and it was now pouring down with rain. I felt discouraged, but I had raised over £250 for the charity behind this event, Cancer Research UK, so I was going to run it no matter what.

At the start line, I felt angry. I think the accumulative emotions of the previous few years had reached a peak inside me and I was just pissed off. Pissed off that we couldn't conceive a baby naturally. Pissed off that IVF hadn't helped us have a successful pregnancy. Pissed off that I had to find ways to occupy myself to take my mind off everything. Pissed off that my husband wasn't well that day. I was just annoyed. I used this anger to push me and I ran faster than I ever had in training. I saw my mum and sister near the end, and seeing them gave me a big boost to run as fast as I could. When I saw the finish line in the distance I wanted to cry. I couldn't believe that I, the previously morbidly obese, sedentary person, was about to finish running a 10k, something I would have thought impossible before. I kept the tears away and crossed the finish line. I took my medal and bottle of water from the volunteer and wandered around. I finished the 10k in fifty-six minutes and I was proud of my achievement.

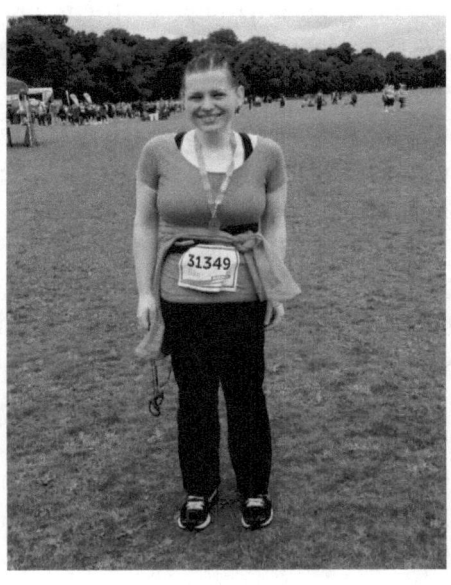

I was elated for the rest of the day. We walked around Cardiff and had a nice lunch and I went home happier than I had been for a long time. I'd already pre-empted the success of this event and had registered for another 10k the weekend after. This time in the other direction geographically, the Llanelli 10k. This time, my mum and my husband came to support me and although I ran it slower, I really enjoyed the scenery and experience. This was more of a running event than a charity event and I relished the atmosphere and drive of the runners around me (mostly in front of me!).

After this event I realised I was hooked. I went home and googled other running events. I'd completed two 10ks, what was next? The Cardiff Half Marathon kept coming up in the search results. 13.1 miles. Could I really do it? Was I fit enough? It was early June at the time and the Cardiff Half wasn't taking place until October, so I figured I had plenty of time to train. Why shouldn't I do it? I'd heard nothing from the clinic, so had no idea when we would be called for our second treatment cycle and I needed something, anything, to focus on. I'd given up on the idea of it happening any time soon. Another event kept catching my eye as well. The Wales Marathon. 26.2 miles. It took place in the summer so it was way too late to train for that kind of distance, but it sat there in my mind, just a little spark saying, 'Wouldn't it be amazing to run a marathon?'

The only negative thing that arose during my successful and continued weight loss was my fixation on the BMI scale. As the BMI is used consistently by medical professionals in the UK, especially for fertility treatment, I had to keep my BMI under thirty in order to still qualify. Once I found the enjoyment in exercise and got used to a new way of eating, this wasn't a problem at all, I was well under thirty and it wasn't a worry. The worry began when realising that even at my smallest (wearing size eight jeans, for example) I was still classified as overweight according to the scale. My BMI never went below twenty-six.

The scale states that below 18.5 is underweight, 18.5 to 24.9 is healthy, 25 to 29.9 is overweight, and over 30 is obese.

I was frustrated that despite looking, feeling and knowing I was a healthy weight and had a good level of fitness, I couldn't seem to be 'officially' healthy according to this chart. I would obsess over this figure and it would nag me in the back of my mind. Perhaps it was merely a diversion from obsessing over our infertility. I would read articles about how inaccurate the scale was since it didn't take into account muscle or body frame, etc., yet I still wasn't happy about it. I had only become acquainted with the BMI scale because of the medical treatment, so if I hadn't known about it and had just lost the weight to get to a point where I felt myself to be healthy, then I would have been thrilled about my current size. But knowing that I was still two numbers away from the healthy section, this chart went from 'you're in the overweight section' to 'you're still fat' in my head and it really wasn't a healthy thing to think about or spend time worrying about.

Part of me wanted to start exercising in an extreme way and cut calories to an unhealthy level just to put my body into the supposed healthy BMI range. But I think the forthcoming treatment cycle saved me from developing a real problem. After all, I needed to be healthy, not undernourished, to be able to have successful treatment. So, despite it living in my head and rearing its ugly head every now and then, I managed to stop it turning into a full-blown obsession. I've since read that the BMI chart has affected a lot of people negatively, making people who would never be able to healthily maintain the suggested weight become obsessed with trying to reach it. I understand that there needs to be some way of measuring what weight is healthy, but surely the medical community should take the chart with a pinch of salt? Surely just looking at someone, or measuring body fat with callipers would make more sense? Maybe even a DEXA scan? (Although I'm sure this is cost prohibitive.) I have a broad shouldered, narrow hipped, muscular physique, and this has an effect on how much I can weigh without becoming obsessive or undernourished to try and get smaller and smaller.

I think we need to have more understanding of the potential inaccuracies of these charts, and realise that just because you've got a BMI that's overweight, it doesn't mean you are. I was once in a room with about twenty fitness trainers, all very fit, muscular and not one of them was actually overweight. Yet none of them had a BMI in the healthy range. They were all 'overweight'. Some of the men were in the early obese section. It just shows that we are the best judge of what is a healthy weight for us individually, not a numerical chart which is archaic and largely unhelpful. Ironically, that chart made me worry more about my weight than I did when I was a hundred and ten pounds heavier.

Along with doing my best to remain positive and attempting to only speak in positive terms about the forthcoming treatment cycle, I had a deck of angel oracle cards, which I would look at most days. I would draw one card from the deck and if it wasn't related to children in some way, I would ignore it. If it was related to children I would take it as a sign that all was well and that our baby was coming to us. On reflection, I was picking cards out with no real question or intention in mind and it felt random.

I also sort of accidentally ended up having a psychic reading at a friend's birthday party. He was a guest but was also happy to do readings if people wanted them. When he saw me he wanted to do a reading straight away (and for no fee). I had never had a face-to-face psychic reading before so I was rather nervous. He knew I'd been through a really tough time and he kept saying that he could see my children, in particular a blonde little girl. During the reading I was quite shocked with the things that were spot on but also dubious about the things which didn't seem right to me. He said that our children were waiting for us and that our treatment would work. I took hope from this and it made me feel better. I ended up going to see him for a proper reading a couple of months later. He was sure the treatment was going to work, and I was more than happy to believe him.

Focused on keeping up my exercise – particularly running for the psychological as well as physical benefits, and having structured, positive goals to work towards, I signed up for the Cardiff Half Marathon and then started my training plan. My husband and I went away on holiday for a week, it was a break we needed. Things were better and we seemed to be coping in a more positive way together, so things were stable.

In total honesty, at this point I was scared to do the second cycle of IVF. I hadn't enjoyed how the drugs had made me feel and I found the whole procedure had taken a massive toll on me physically and mentally. There was so much extra pressure this time too – this was our second and final cycle, if this didn't work it would be the end of the road for us. We would have to face a childless life together and neither of us was ready or willing to explore that scenario at that point in time.

It was the middle of the summer when the letter finally arrived in the post to let us know that our second IVF treatment cycle would begin with my next menstrual cycle. A mix of anticipation, excitement and trepidation consumed us both. The treatment itself was difficult, and I knew that I could only get through it again if there was a positive outcome.

This time we had to be successful. It had to bring us our baby.

Chapter Six
Give it one more go

The summer was drawing to a close when the treatment cycle started. I had the usual consultations, started the Norethisterone, and then moved on to the down-regulating injections exactly the same as last time. I was still running but had come to the conclusion that I wouldn't be able to do the Cardiff Half Marathon, as I would hopefully be in early pregnancy by early October, and I wouldn't have felt comfortable. But I kept running as I felt it was good for my mental health. I decided that I'd stop once I started the follicle stimulating hormone injections, as I thought that rest would be preferable and wise at that point. I was quite sad to not be able to run a half marathon after following the training plan so diligently, so I just continued, knowing that I'd stop before long. I figured that I'd get pregnant with this treatment cycle and then a half marathon would be on the back burner for quite some time.

However, I then had the idea to run my own half marathon on the cycle path local to me, instead of doing the official half marathon. I even decided to raise more money for charity and split the money raised (about £170) between three charities

(Barnardo's, Cats Protection and the John Hartson Foundation), which seemed to make it feel more official to me and it was a push to keep up my training. One day in September, I headed out to run my first half marathon. I had mapped the route previously and was using an app on my phone to count the miles as well, making it as accurate as I possibly could. All was going well. It was a nice morning and I felt good. I don't know whether it was because it wasn't such a shock this time or whether my body was more used to the drugs, but I wasn't feeling as bad during this section of the treatment. Overall, I seemed to be dealing with the treatment better this time around. I'd read a few articles online about how keeping up the exercise was beneficial to the treatment's outcome, and I had the agreement of my consultant to keep running during this section of treatment. About five miles into the run, I very desperately needed a pee. This had never happened to me before (and happily never has since) but I had to go. It was find a place to do it discreetly or wet my pants. I ended up squatting in some bushes, praying no one would come along. I was mortified. I have since learnt that getting caught short while out running is quite a common scenario, but it certainly wasn't common for me! I can only assume that I'd panic drunk too much water before leaving the house.

It wasn't a fast half marathon by any means, about two hours forty-seven minutes in total, but that didn't matter to me. When I passed the 13.1-mile mark I walked the rest of the way home and I was overwhelmed with the achievement. I couldn't believe just how far I had come. When I got back to the house I immediately showered and reflected on all I had managed to achieve between the two treatment cycles, despite the heartbreak – maybe even because of the heartbreak. I felt a bit proud of myself for the first time in a long time.

It wasn't much longer before I was starting the Menopur

injections again. The dose was somewhere between the initial and upped dose of the last cycle, so I hoped that this would make some kind of difference to the outcome. Aside from the local clinic being fully functional at this point and the location being completely different, the cycle itself was practically identical. I was clinging onto any positivity and hope I could find, listing reasons to be grateful and repeating positive affirmations to try and keep my mindset from dwelling on all the things that could go wrong. After all, this was our last chance; it had to work. It had to.

I had read about people using alternative therapies to complement their treatment, particularly acupuncture. I wasn't super keen on this idea at first. I hadn't considered any alternative therapies to run alongside our treatment for our first cycle, but after the outcome of the first cycle and my faith being shaken up, I was more willing to give it a go. I'd had one session of reflexology which was actually a lovely and calm experience, so I thought why not try acupuncture? I had nothing to lose by trying it. I found an acupuncturist who seemed ideal and I emailed her all my information about my treatment cycle, so that she would understand my delicate situation. I ended up having two sessions with this lady and my husband had one. I didn't get off to the best start with her as she hadn't bothered to read any of the IVF information I had emailed her ahead of time, so I had to explain it all to her during the session, which I was just so tired of doing in general. She asked me questions that I found frustrating, but I gave her the benefit of the doubt and had the first treatment.

This was during the down-regulation stage, before I ran the half marathon. I think my husband and I both felt like we'd had a little pick-me-up after the experience, so I went back to see her for a further session when I was deep into the follicle stimulating injection phase. My stomach was all bruised up from the many, many injections so it didn't seem like more needles would matter. I had the second treatment, and if nothing else it was helpful for me to have a bit of time to just relax. But secretly I hoped that this would be the miracle thing that would make this treatment a success.

At one of the ultrasound scans it was noted that I seemed to have responded well to the Menopur and didn't need a dosage change this time, so I was booked in for my egg collection. This time we didn't have to travel, it could all be done at the local clinic. It was brand new, with the latest technology; everything was in our favour. The consultant proudly spoke of how we wouldn't find a better clinic anywhere else. I remember doing the final injection of hCG and feeling a bit shaky with expectation. I'd done everything I could now, every injection, every appointment, everything I'd been told to do. I had bought cheap pregnancy tests in bulk so that I could test each day after the hCG injection – so that I could watch the test go from positive (due to the hCG injection) to negative to positive again (due to pregnancy causing the hCG hormone). I had seen people document this online, watching the line go from bright, to faint, to gone, to faint to bright again. I remember looking at the result of the first test and noting that it was a very weak positive, but as the tests themselves were cheap, I thought little more of it – perhaps the tests just didn't have a lot of dye.

The day arrived to head back to the clinic and I couldn't stop myself from feeling very scared. It felt like everything was riding on this procedure and the pressure was just too great. The procedure would be exactly the same as last time with regards to how they collected the eggs; the only difference was I was only going to be sedated, not given a general anaesthetic. My husband went off to provide his sperm sample and I had to go and insert suppositories – I honestly cannot remember what they were for now. I went back to sit on my bed and my husband returned not long after. The nurse gave him a sarcastic look as if to say, 'Oh well done, your bit done now? Must have been difficult for you...'

We sat there making quiet conversation until someone came over to insert a cannula into the top of my hand, but for some reason they couldn't do it properly. This went on so long that a nurse realised that I was going to faint, so ordered me to lie down while she sorted out the cannula. I was starting to get impatient now, so was relieved when I was finally wheeled into the theatre and given the drug for sedation. This egg collection was a lot more stressful than the first. I was sedated so I was awake, but everything was a bit fuzzy and weird and I couldn't keep track of time. I was lying down on the bed in the theatre with my legs propped open and my new consultant guiding a needle up through my vagina. I remember feeling pain and discomfort.

While this was going on I swear about a hundred different people seemed to go in and out of the room. 'Oh hi! Come on in, take a good look, the more the merrier!' One thing is for sure, after IVF treatment you'll never worry about a smear test again. Every now and then my consultant would say something to me, probably just updating me on what he was doing, how long was left, that sort of thing. When it was over he said he'd collected five eggs. I was too out of it to really think about the number but I obviously realised that it was half the number of the last cycle.

After I was left to recover on the ward with a coffee and some biscuits, they wheeled in another woman. She was very vocal and, I noticed straight away, very negative. I listened to her go on about how it wasn't going to work anyway, how the whole thing was pointless, and how caffeine caused miscarriages so how dare the staff offer her tea or coffee. She was blatantly not thinking about anyone other than herself or the fear or negativity she was putting into my mind or anyone else's. My husband and I kept glancing at each other awkwardly while she continued on with her rant. I remember a nurse trying to calm her down. I kept thinking, well I'm positive that this is going to work. Five eggs – it must be quality over quantity this time. But the woman was just scared and that was the only way she knew how to deal with it.

After I'd been there for the required recovery time, the embryologist came to speak to us. He went over the information, confirmed that they had five eggs to work with and that he would ring me tomorrow to let me know what had happened and what was going to happen. We went home, rested, and pinned all our hopes on this being the miracle we needed.

The next morning my husband went off to work as normal and I stayed home and watched some mindless television programmes. I noticed the hours going by and thought it was strange that the embryologist hadn't rung in the morning. They definitely rang me in the morning last time. But it was okay, I knew all was well. After all, no news is good news, right? Finally, in the afternoon my mobile rang and I had just enough signal for the call, so I answered eagerly. It was the embryologist, and somehow just from the way he greeted me I felt my body freeze. He said he was sorry but he wasn't ringing with good news. Without another word I felt my whole world crash down around me.

Of the five eggs only two had been suitable for attempted insemination. They'd tried injecting the two eggs with sperm but one of the eggs had cracked and the other had just not fertilised. It seemed that they were coated with a hard layer and there had been nothing they could do achieve fertilisation. He said they could tell when they'd been collected that something wasn't right with them but they tried to inseminate them anyway just in case. I said nothing but the required utterances needed for a formal conversation. He told me that he would book us in for a review meeting with the consultant and then apologised again before ending the phone call. I put the phone down on the cushion next to me and tried to find a way of calming myself, but it wasn't possible. I'd gone through this mindfuck treatment twice now only to be left with nothing. Every injection, every procedure had been an utter waste of time.

When I say my world crashed down around me, I mean that everything shattered. My faith, my strength, everything. It was all broken. I was suffocating with tears and I felt as if the walls were closing in on me and I couldn't breathe. Everything was dark. It was all over and no dreams were ever coming true.

CHAPTER SEVEN
When IVF fails

Some things that suck when you're an infertile woman:

1. That conversation when you meet new people:

'So do you have kids?'

'No.'

'Why?'

'My reproductive organs are ineffective.'

'...'

2. When people say stuff around you like: 'Oh, having kids is just the best thing ever.' 'My life just wasn't complete until we had a baby.' 'The greatest thing I've done with my life is have children.' Awkward.

3. When everyone around you is having babies and you spend lots of time shopping for baby presents and pretend it doesn't bother you that it's always for other people.

4. When people have no idea what it's like to suffer from infertility

and they make stupid comments.

'How is it possible that IVF didn't work?'

'What's wrong with you?'

'Stop trying and it'll happen!'

'I dunno how I would cope with life if I didn't have my kids.' (Great, thanks.)

'Just relax!'

'Can't you just have more fertility treatment?' (Are you gonna pay for it for me?)

'Haven't you thought about adoption?' (Do you know I hadn't! I'll pop down the orphanage on the weekend and pick a cute one...)

'You'll never push a baby out of those hips!' (Sorry, what?)

5. Reaching an age where it becomes socially unacceptable to not have children. 'Yeah, she's in her thirties, been married years and NO KIDS... yeah, so weird... must be something wrong with her.'

6. Facebook announcements and scan photos. As happy as you are for them it still tears you up inside as you don't get to experience it. And THAT comment: 'Now we're a REAL family.'

7. When friends drift away as their lives are now all about their kids and you have no common ground anymore.

8. Going through fertility treatment and it doesn't work for you.

9. When super-fertile people tell you that they fall pregnant without even trying. (What do you want? A freaking medal?)

10. When people try and make you feel better by telling you kids are a pain in the ass and you're lucky not to have them. Or they offer you theirs: 'You can have mine if you want.'

11. When you want to seem positive and not bitter but fail miserably.

I still remember that phone call from the embryologist so clearly, even today. I remember the sheer helplessness and fear and overwhelming nightmarish feelings it provoked. Not only was this dream over with nowhere to go – we simply didn't have the money for a further cycle – but all the pain had been for nothing. So what do you do when you've reached the end of the road? What do you do when IVF fails? It's supposed to create a miracle, isn't it? Well where was our miracle? Did we not deserve one?

I had to phone my husband and ask him to come home from work. Of course, I didn't want to tell him what had happened over the phone, but I'd just been told it over the phone so I didn't know what else to do. He, of course, wanted to know what had happened immediately. I cried and cried and cried and cried. Not only was our dream shattered, but my faith in everything was destroyed. My beliefs, my positive thinking, my hope, it was gone with that dream. I didn't know how I could hold onto it. I couldn't see a way. I know my husband felt broken over this as well.

One of the hardest things was having to tell everyone that the treatment had failed so early on in the process. I had to deal with people asking how it was even possible for it to fail at that point. People now seemed to understand that with IVF miscarriages can happen, that embryos don't always implant properly and that no pregnancy might occur, but they couldn't understand how after all that treatment, my eggs could be of such a pathetic quality that they couldn't handle being injected by a single sperm. And I didn't know what to say. It just hadn't worked. I felt like the dark clouds had started raining and there was no rainbow in sight, it just poured down on my head and I was soaked to the skin.

It took me several days to feel like I could properly function again, albeit with difficulty. My body was messed up from all the hormones and the procedure and I just felt barren. Void of life. And now I had to go back to my life and back to work and back to acting like it was okay. 'Just wasn't meant to be, I suppose.' And deal with people's confusion and pity. I felt like I'd written a script and would repeat it verbatim whenever talking to anyone. Several times I was asked how much a further cycle would cost and when I responded with the amount, it would end the conversation. A few stories were repeated to us about how they knew someone who had IVF and it didn't work and then they ended up getting pregnant naturally anyway, but that sort of story just couldn't shine any light on the darkness at that time. I was quite frankly lost. It was almost the end of September and if I wanted to, I could still take part in the Cardiff Half Marathon, the first weekend in October, but that seemed laughable. I kept dwelling on everything over and over, thinking about our journey from start to finish again and again. I couldn't cope with having my faith destroyed along with my dream; I really didn't know what to think.

It all starts so simply, you decided to try to get pregnant or you stop taking birth control with a 'we'll see what happens' attitude. Then all of a sudden it's another month, another negative test, another agonising wait for the blood to start so you can restart and begin another month of regimented fucking. And your hormones are raging, you're devastated and angry AGAIN.

You decide to go on Facebook for a nose, and oh what's that? Another fucking scan photo. And another one. We're expecting! And you're not... you're not expecting. You're not expecting this month, or last month or any of the other bloody months you've been having unprotected sex trying to catch the mystical ovulation with several million of your partner's sperm. And even treatment doesn't work for you! Oh dear. Someone else's joy has turned you cold and bitter and you cry. Then you force yourself to leave a sickly sweet comment on the photo while you lose yourself in the unfairness of it all.

But you're not a bad person, you don't mean to think badly or want to tear up their joy. It's just they've gone and achieved the thing you want more than anything in the world. But life is denying you the experience and it's a reminder, it's yet another reminder that you've failed. And you're not evil, you are happy for them, but you just have to process the information differently at the moment. And then the guilt arrives because you think you're a horrible, selfish person.

The people on the TTC forum understand, they get it. But then one by one they get up the duff as well and soon you're in the TTC 1+ year group, then the TTC 2+ year group, then you're in the IVF group and then you're nowhere as there's nowhere else to go once IVF has failed.

In truth, I often felt selfish for being so upset, for feeling so depressed. There were so many awful things going on in the world, so many awful things happening to other people. I felt like I was ignoring all the good in my life and focusing on the pain too much, despite attempts at doing the opposite. But I didn't know how to change it, because this was my world and the only one I knew at that time. This is not just isolated to infertility. Whatever is causing your world to crash down or perpetuate low mood is overwhelming to you personally and it's difficult to compare with other people's problems because you only have experience of your own, not everyone else's as well. You can't sit there and create a hierarchy of heartbreak, and if yours isn't as bad as others then not allow yourself to feel upset over it, it doesn't work like that. You can sympathise and feel terrible, but you can't live other people's pain. You can only live your own pain and no matter what it is, it can be earth shattering. And sometimes people won't understand how you feel because unless they've been through infertility or depression or whatever then it can be hard to understand. If you haven't been through it, you just don't know.

We had our appointment letter for our review with the consultant in the post soon after the phone call with the embryologist. I don't think either of us saw any point in attending this – we couldn't have any more treatment with them, so what was the man going to say to us? We couldn't afford any more treatment anywhere. But we decided to go, perhaps it would be the closure we needed. On the morning of the appointment, the motorway traffic was horrendous and we, and everyone else, were late for our appointments. By the time we were sitting in the waiting room I was already stressed and on the verge of tears. My husband had to get back to work and time was ticking on and on. I asked the receptionist a few times how much longer it would be. The final time I asked, I lost it and said I didn't see what the point of us being there was.

They must have realised how distressed I was because they alerted the consultant immediately and he practically came straight out. Apparently, he had been busy familiarising himself with our notes. We went into his consulting room and told him we only had fifteen minutes before we had to leave. I asked him if there was much point in having this consultation, but he encouraged us to stay and offered me a tissue to wipe my face, as I was very emotional. We went over what went wrong with our cycle. My eggs weren't of a good quality; my husband's sperm sample was very poor. Yes, we had figured that out for ourselves. He told us not to be too despondent and explained that fertility goes up and down. Eggs are not necessarily always of a suitable quality to be fertilised and that was normal and natural. He said that one month they might be good and the next month not so good, it was the way of our bodies and they couldn't do much about that. I understood what he was saying but it didn't help to heal the feeling of failure raging within me.

He encouraged us to have more treatment if we could afford it. He said we would be better off seeking treatment abroad as it would be cheaper. I was listening to him but I knew I would never undertake another IVF cycle. As much as I wanted children, I had found the process too emotionally and physically difficult. I felt like the two cycles had taken their toll on my body and aged me and I just wanted to heal now. I thought about women who just kept going until they had a successful cycle and while I admired their tenacity and resilience, I just knew I couldn't do it. As much as it hurt to accept we would never be able to have our own biological children, I knew I couldn't cope with facing this treatment again. Perhaps I would have felt differently if we'd had the money for further treatment and I could have approached the situation in an entirely different manner. But we didn't and we didn't want to go bankrupt getting loan after loan to fund it. I mentioned adoption and the consultant stated that adoption was harder than IVF. Yes, emotionally it would be, but at least I wouldn't be undertaking treatment physically. We knew then and there that adoption would be our next step when we were ready to consider it.

On the way home from our review appointment, I pondered the

opinion that some people seem to have – that the doctors are playing God in the lab and creating life during IVF treatment. I have come to the very firm conclusion that this is not the case. Life isn't being created in the lab; life is being given assistance, a helping hand. The two elements are helped to get together and develop into an embryo or blastocyst but they cannot force it to become life. You can have top quality eggs and sperm together and fertilisation still won't take place; or it will only to then fail and not develop, or fail to implant. Life decides whether it wants to be created or not, not us.

All the clinic appointments were now over, and aside from the forthcoming sessions with the infertility counsellor, there was now nothing to tie us to the clinic or the treatment. That part of life was finished. I really wasn't sure what to do now. Or how to feel. Infertility and treatment had been the focus of our lives for such a long time that there was now a gaping hole which needed to be filled, or we risked being pulled into the blackness. Reality was now setting in but I still felt a lot of numbness over everything. I couldn't quite understand how everything I believed in had let me down. It seemed that no amount of positive thinking or prayer could've changed the outcome. But I needed to do something, anything, to put myself on a path to healing.

Over the past year I had made a couple of impulsive decisions, like signing up for the 10k despite never running before, and I wanted to do something else which would require a structured programme, focus and dedication, something I could really give myself to. Nothing I could think of was quite right, other than maybe a marathon… or two? I had to move on. I had to find a way. So, merely a week or so after the phone call with the embryologist, I signed up for the Wales Marathon (taking place the following summer) and I had contacted several children's charities to see if I could run for them for the London Marathon. It seemed a bit premature and crazy, but I was looking for something big to distract me and to help me move on and be part of my healing. Nothing but a big gesture would do.

I still had my race number for the Cardiff Half Marathon. It had arrived in the post weeks before and I had held onto it because I didn't know what else to do with it. It seemed wrong to just throw it away. The event was over a week away and I needed something to think about that had nothing to do with treatment or infertility or babies. So I made the snap decision to take part. A few people questioned this decision. Physically, I wasn't ready, and who knew about my mental state? I wouldn't be able to run it all as the treatment had battered my fitness level, but I could run and walk and I could make it to the end, I just knew I could.

After making this decision, I received an email from the running co-ordinator at The Children's Trust, one of the charities I had contacted, saying that they wanted me on their London Marathon team for April next year. I was going to run the London Marathon. Me. I felt the excitement rise up within me, something that I'd feared I would never experience again.

Chapter Eight
Rebuilding

On the first Sunday in October 2013, I got up very early and tiptoed out of my house to make the journey to Cardiff for the half marathon. I decided to go by myself I'm not entirely sure why exactly but I knew that my husband (who was not a fan of crowds anyway) would benefit more from having rest at home than to stand around for hours waiting for me to finish. In less than a week I had raised £245 for the charity Barnardo's. I thought it was a positive thing to do and something which would make me feel useful again. I parked my car in the usual place but sat in the car for ages, watching other runners park up and head towards the area by the start line. Gosh, they all looked fit – much fitter than me. I'd gained some weight during the IVF cycle (almost identically to the first cycle) and my fitness had suffered greatly in a short time, so I was concerned at how I would make it through the 13.1 miles without significant periods of walking, but that wasn't going to put me off. Not today.

I finally mustered up the courage to get myself out of the car and, of course, I headed straight to the toilets to take several nervous wees. I had pinned my race number on my running vest in the car, and I had everything I needed in my running belt, so technically I was ready to go. I had run this distance not so long ago, but that was at home, on paths I knew well, with no time limits, before the rest of the injections and egg collection, with no one watching. This was a new experience. This was a big event. The two 10k events I'd done previously were very small events, nothing like this. I went to find my starting pen, somewhere close to the back, and looked around. I didn't seem quite so out of place after all, there were people of all shapes and sizes there, everyone in different colours, smiling and happy. Perhaps I'd been worrying unnecessarily. And it didn't matter if I had, it was a relief to worry and think about something that wasn't related to infertility for once! I ended up queuing for the portaloos for one final pee before going back to my pen for the start. My experience in the bushes from the first half marathon had made me a tad paranoid.

The event began and because I was so close to the back it took a while to get to the starting line, but once I crossed it I started running. I ran the first mile as best I could in my current state and I didn't stop. I was a couple of miles into it before I took my first walking break and from then on I switched between running and walking. There wasn't support present on the entire route but there were areas where people had crowded together to cheer, and that was encouraging. It was uplifting to see people cheering everyone on. It was nice to see people running in costumes and charity vests and I was thoroughly distracted by everything for the first five or six miles.

Then about halfway through it started to hurt a little, and then the doubt about whether or not I could finish it, crept in. Running is often a psychological battle between your body and your mind. But you just have to push through. Suddenly, I was thinking about everything – infertility, the miscarriage, the failed

IVF, that we would never have children. But these thoughts weren't sending me to a dark place, I was still going forward, still in the race. I was working through all of this stuff in my head as I ran/walked. I was going over everything and asking myself questions. Why would I hold onto the belief that it was going to happen only for it to fail so spectacularly? Why would I find this place of positivity and faith only to have it all tested in this way? Why couldn't the timing have been right? Why couldn't my body have worked better? Why couldn't I at least have made one quality egg? Was I not meant to have children? Had I been barking up the wrong tree the whole time? It went on and on like this and, of course, I felt emotional, but I kept going. How do I move on from this? How do I find a way to forge a new type of life for myself? How do I leave all this hurt and sorrow behind me? Just keep going. I asked God to show me the way, to help me find a way through this. I still didn't know how, other than to keep going.

One thing that has annoyingly always stuck with me from that event, was a comment from an arrogant spectator near the halfway point. I don't know why, but I heard him clear as day. 'Look at them, not even halfway and they're all exhausted. Haha.' I've never wanted to stop and yell at someone more than in that moment. If you're not going to be encouraging, then shut the fuck up. It's easy to judge when you're standing there and not taking part. I hoped that no one else had heard him. I could cope with moving forward in the face of criticism, as it certainly wasn't the worst thing to happen of late, but I didn't know if those around me could.

About three miles from the end, I had pretty much stopped running. I was giving a little effort now and then but I was exhausted and just wanted to walk. Sometimes you find the most strength in the tail end of events because you'll meet people and speak to people and get each other through it. I was talking to a lady who was raising money for a children's cancer hospital and she was struggling to make it through, so we encouraged each other for the last couple of miles. I remember seeing so many people walking in the opposite direction to us, medal around their neck, race t-shirt on, goodie bag in hand and I thought 'that'll be me soon, I'm so close'. As I finally saw the finish line ahead I ran over it; there was a little boost of energy hidden in me somewhere so I used it. I had done it. I had kept going even when I didn't think I could.

That's the thing about running, you learn more about yourself during an event than you ever expected. It took me three hours and thirteen minutes to cross that finish line and I'd been through a psychological journey as well as a physical one. But I'd successfully set a tone for who I wanted to be and what I wanted to achieve, and that really was a light which illuminated the darkness.

Just keep going. That's all I had to do.

Later that month it was my thirtieth birthday. Initially, I didn't want to do anything at all to celebrate, it seemed pointless when I was dealing with so much pain below the surface all the time. But luckily one of my friends took charge of it and we planned a Harry Potter party. I knew that if I was going to have a party I wanted it to be childlike. What better way was there to turn thirty? I was done with being an adult and was ready to regress for the night. I had quite a few friends to stay and it was refreshing to spend time with friends in a carefree and happy manner. We dressed up as if we were part of the wizarding world and just enjoyed our butterbeer and cupcakes. It was a welcome break.

We hadn't actually been social or seen many people other than work colleagues and medical professionals through the treatment cycle, so as a couple we really had been in our own little world – an IVF bubble, you could say. I know a lot of people have a bit of a crisis about turning thirty, as if it's the end of youth and the reality of age becomes apparent to them. I didn't feel like that at all. I felt the scariest thing had already happened to me the previous month, so turning thirty had no real significance other than the fact that I was starting a new age decade. In many ways, it seemed organised to leave all the treatment and struggles behind with my twenties and move forward into my thirties with a different focus. Of course, it wasn't that simple, but if nothing else at least the physical side of all the treatment and infertility had been left in my twenties.

I started to see the infertility counsellor at the hospital a couple of days after my birthday. Initially, my husband and I attended together, but then I went to see her alone. I changed over the course of these sessions. In the very first appointment I was a mess, crying and unsure what I was now meant to do with my life. But slowly I saw myself becoming stronger. It was refreshing to talk to someone about it, someone who knew what to say in response and knew the right questions to ask. The 'right questions' are as individual as the experience itself. The important thing is to listen and just be there for the person. Ask them how they are, really listen to their response, and go from there.

The counsellor helped me identify ways to move forward and challenged my fixation on failure. All of the things I felt I should have achieved and hadn't were personal, familial and societal pressures, and in truth I didn't have to achieve any of them. It wasn't essential for a recently turned thirty-year-old to worry about or seek any of it. These expectations were weights tied to my legs, weighing me down in the water making me unable to move. However, from the shore you could only see my top half so the weights weren't visible. One by one, I had to untangle myself or cut myself free and swim away. I didn't have a huge number of sessions with the counsellor, and after a few weeks I had been completely discharged, but it was constructive while it lasted. Now there was no visible connection whatsoever to everything we had been through over the years.

It really was time to move on. I had marathons to train for, I had plans to make for my career and my education. I was volunteering for charities, I was fundraising, I was working, I was doing everything I could to find a way to move forward. I threw myself into anything and everything that came along. On reflection I was spreading myself too thin but anything that took the focus away from infertility was more than welcome in my life.

Chapter Nine
Refocus

I had made this massive commitment and now I actually had to go through with it. I'd meticulously planned my training, with progression each week and appropriate rest periods. It was seventeen weeks long and due to start in December. I even had a treadmill now (thirtieth birthday present) so that I could train indoors if I needed to. I had also started my fundraising. I was determined to smash my £1800 target. I was still dealing with the aftermath of IVF and I found that it seemed to hit me in waves. Still, this new focus was a great step forward. I was attempting to turn my pain into positivity.

The first week of my training plan looked like this –

Day 1: 3 mile run (easy run)

Day 2: Circuit training

Day 3: 7 mile run (long run)

Day 4: 3 mile run (mix of easy/steady running)

Day 5: Circuit training

Day 6: 3 mile run (steady run)

Day 7: rest day

And it progressed week by week until my longest run become twenty-two miles.

I loved the first week of the training plan, it just felt awesome to be following something structured again. It helped keep me focused and appealed to my goal-orientated nature. At that time I was utilising the treadmill a lot because I was still a little self-conscious after gaining weight during the last IVF cycle and the weather was typical for that time of year, so the only outdoors runs at that time were the longer ones. I remember really enjoying my long run during that first week. It was one of those lovely runs where you felt like you could just keep running. I noticed that my speed was improving – I wasn't fast but I was starting to see improvements again. It was pleasing to me and it was uplifting. I was updating my blog regularly and I found that it was a really great tool for staying on track as well.

I was really committed to raising money for my charity. I chose The Children's Trust, as they did amazing work for children with brain injuries, multiple disabilities and complex health needs, and supported their families too. In fact, I reached the halfway point in my fundraising before Christmas, so I was doing really well. People were supportive and generous and I was doing my best to think up ways to generate sponsorship (one idea in particular was a cookbook raffle).

Aside from running and volunteering and fundraising and working and all the other things I had taken on, we decided that it was finally time to move. We were fed up with where we were living and the house just had too many unhappy memories. We decided we wanted to move further west, about an hour away, to a coastal area with good routes for running and walking. But we didn't know how we would manage it, we just had to wait and see how it would all work out.

I found Christmas to be a difficult time as it's primarily aimed towards children, and we didn't have any and wouldn't be having any, so it was hard. The Christmas parade came and went and I didn't attend. That wish hadn't come true – I didn't have a baby to take with me. I decided to head out on a long run on Christmas morning, as I wanted to take the focus away from everything I lacked and think about everything I had to gain. At the very least the endorphins from my run improved the day immeasurably. As we got further away from the treatment, I started to consider adoption more and more. I knew it would be difficult, but I thought that maybe towards the end of the year it might be something we could consider. But at that point it wasn't something that we were ready to discuss. Instead I trained diligently and despite the usual setbacks (stomach bug, a cold, a bad week, that sort of thing) it was all going really well and I was feeling better than I had done for a long time.

In early 2014 I started to question the benefit of continuing to take Metformin, the drug I'd been prescribed when I'd first received my PCOS diagnosis. I didn't feel that it had really helped and now that our fertility treatment was over with there seemed even less point in continuing with it. I visited my local general practitioner to seek their approval for discontinuing the drug but frustratingly I was told that the decision would have to be made by my consultant. I explained that I had already been discharged so there was no consultant for me to ask, but that seemed to mean nothing. So I left that appointment perturbed to have been left in a sort of limbo, and had to make the decision myself instead. I stopped taking the drug immediately and I haven't returned to it since.

In early March, I ran my first official half marathon of the year (I was up to eighteen miles on my training plan, and those eighteen miles had been a real mental and physical struggle). It was the Llanelli Half Marathon in West Wales. I was really excited for this event, as it was the first event where I felt properly prepared – or as prepared as I could really be at that point. I still wasn't particularly quick but I had the endurance to keep going with minimal discomfort now. I'd lost the weight from the last IVF and I was feeling comfortable. The start was at the Parc Y Scarlets Stadium, and as I'd experienced already, I went for about five nervous wees before heading to the start line. My mum came to support me despite the stormy conditions. It was a very scenic course but also very windy and rainy in portions. I loved it. I enjoyed reading the backs of the other runners' vests to see which club they had come from or what charity they were supporting.

It was a 'there and back' course so once I was on the heading back portion I was really feeling like I could do it. It was entirely different to how I felt doing the Cardiff Half the previous year. I wasn't struggling through, I wasn't going over and over things in my head, I was just allowing myself to be, as I watched the scenery go by. It was almost like meditation, although certainly a more physically brutal meditation! When I saw the stadium on the right hand side as I ran the final mile I saw my mum and some other runners I had spoken to at the start (who had already finished) standing there behind the barrier cheering me on and I really was excited and happy. I threw my hands in the air. I had almost done it. I didn't care how long it had taken me, I was just thrilled. I saw the finish line as I turned the last corner and I felt that final hit of energy to sprint across the line. I finished in two hours and thirty-three minutes, a whole forty minutes faster than the Cardiff Half. This was real progression and I was experiencing it.

Training continued, and a couple of weeks later I was heading back to Llanelli to take part in the HBA 5-10-20. It was a small event and you could choose to run five, ten or twenty miles. I had decided to do the twenty-mile version as it fitted in well with my training for London. For some reason, I hadn't made myself aware of the route beforehand, which was probably a good thing as I might not have taken part if I had. The first half was up hill and the second half back down. I started off feeling pretty good; there were still other people from the other distances alongside me so I wasn't feeling isolated or too slow. I ran strongly for miles. I started to lose the will a little as I was approaching the turning point at mile ten and realised that there was no one running with me. I'd seen everyone making their way back down as I was still climbing up and I was sure I was the last person – something I hadn't experienced before.

The route was pretty most of the time, so that was a welcome distraction, but my head was full of self-doubt. As I reached the turning point I stopped to chat to the volunteers who were manning the point. They told me I wasn't the final person because there was no one on a bike behind me. They asked me whether I was fundraising as well and I told them about The Children's Trust and the work the charity does. As I was running off, one of the volunteers told me to just think of the children and I would get through it. On the way back down I saw the final two runners with the sweeper bike behind them and we exchanged encouraging words as we passed. I felt strong again for a few miles, but I was still taking walking breaks every so often. At one point, I stopped to walk with a lady who was walking her dog, as she wanted to know more about the event. I wasn't concerned about my finishing time, I was just happy to get to the end.

Then around mile fourteen, I hit what I assume people refer to as 'the wall'. I kept telling myself that I just couldn't do it.

I wouldn't finish. I couldn't run the twenty miles today and I couldn't do the marathon either. The whole thing was worthless and pointless and I hated myself and everything. Very dramatic, I know, but if a sweeper van had gone past (or even the man with his bike) I would have hopped on and headed straight to the finish. I went over everything that had happened and felt like everything was my fault. I felt like all my attempts at being positive and moving on were ridiculous. I remember seeing piles of water bottles at mile markers but no one manning the spots anymore – I had taken so long that it seemed the volunteers had given up and gone home.

This mental torment carried on until I saw the sign for mile seventeen, and despite now being so close to the end, my head was done. I was on the easiest part of the course and I only had three miles to go but I was losing the mental battle. I genuinely didn't think I could do it and in total honesty I cried, but I made myself keep walking. Then I thought of what the volunteer had said to me – think of the children. And I started running again and I didn't stop until I ran straight across the finish line, hands in the air, big smile on my face. I'd had it in me after all – I just didn't know how to access it. I had faced the most difficult and long-lasting mental battle I'd ever experienced while running and I'd smashed straight through it. I could do this. I finished at four hours eleven minutes, 103rd out of 105 runners (for the twenty miler) and I felt that if I could get through that, I could get through anything.

I remember talking about this event with friends afterwards, and the general consensus was that if I could do this hilly twenty miler, London would be no problem at all. Yes, it had 6.2 extra miles, but they were at least flat miles. It gave me a boost to think about it that way. I just hoped they were right, because if I didn't manage to cross the finish line in London it would be a huge disappointment. And I was fed up of disappointment. I was preoccupied with the marathon and training and fundraising, but that didn't stop me from daydreaming about becoming pregnant or dwelling on the past. I would be having a super positive day and then for whatever reason the topic of pregnancy/children would come up and I'd feel all the pain slowly rise to the surface.

The worst was when I'd meet someone new and they'd ask if I had children, to which I would answer no. 'Do you have children?' is the question that hits you right in the stomach. Then they'd ask if I wanted children, and depending on how I was feeling that day my answer would change. Some days I'd say 'hopefully one day' and other days I'd just say 'actually we can't have children' and cue the awkward moment. It was like when the rain rests in droplets on blades of grass so delicately, but all it takes is something to quietly brush past to cause it all to fall. Sometimes I would find myself talking candidly about it all, keeping all the hurt below the surface and everything visible looking calm and amenable. But it's a loaded question. Though it might be asked innocently, people do need to be aware that they might not get a simple answer in response. There are so many reasons why someone might want children but not have them and by asking the innocent yet invasive question you could be causing them to relive things they are trying to put behind them or upsetting them. It's hard enough when pregnancy and babies are already everywhere so when the question is direct to you, it makes it so much more difficult to pretend you're okay. When my husband started a new job there was a morning meeting with the entire branch present and someone asked him if he was married, he said yes. Next question was, 'Do you have kids?' And he said no. Next question was, 'Why?' He wasn't ready to put up his deflective armour at that moment so he simply said that he would rather not talk about it. But the response to 'no I don't have children' should never be 'why?' – it really is inappropriate.

After the twenty-mile event I was heading into tapering, so the long runs were getting drastically shorter to provide rest before the marathon which was now only a few weeks away. I found myself swinging between sheer excitement and crippling nerves. This was really significant to me. In all my years of obesity and being unfit I could never have believed I was going to run a marathon, and the London Marathon no less! I'd watched a time-lapse video which showed the full 26.2 miles. I was utterly in awe of it.

The opportunity arose to take part in the Yeovil Half Marathon and despite previously deciding that I wouldn't do anymore organised events before the big day, I couldn't resist. The atmosphere, the social aspect and the chance to get another medal was too big a temptation. There were three reasons why this was the perfect last event to do before London. The first being an excuse to make a new friend (a running buddy from the online running club I belonged to had kindly offered to provide lunch and cake after the race). The second being that my long run for the coming weekend needed to be thirteen miles, so a half marathon was ideal. The third and probably the most significant was because the previous year I happened to be driving through Yeovil on the day of the half marathon, and at that point I hadn't started running. I remember thinking about how much I wanted to run and take part in events like this. Everyone else said things along the lines of 'Imagine running this today? No, thank you! How awful!' and I nodded along but inside I really wanted to be one of the runners. This was what I really wanted to do with my Sundays, with or without children. So it seemed that taking part in this event would be the perfect acknowledgement of how far I'd come.

Not being familiar with the area at all, I managed to get totally lost trying to find the start of the half marathon. I was driving around and just getting more and more confused and consumed with the clock ticking. I didn't want to miss the event. In total honesty, I have no idea how I ended up finding the place in the end, I think the angels must have been smiling on me and just showed me the right way to go because I still don't know how I managed to get unlost. I parked the car, threw everything I needed in my running belt and legged it down to towards the starting line.

Of course, I needed the toilet. And, of course, there was a queue – mainly full of people who weren't actually running. Faced with nothing but blocked toilets, I couldn't help but be reminded of my husband's experience at the hospital. Luckily I found someone official-looking to let them know about the nightmare in the cubicles before heading towards the starting line. At the last minute before the event started, I recognised my new friend and we arranged where we would meet afterwards (she was considerably faster than me so we wouldn't be running together). I joined the people towards the back and about a minute or so later we were off. Who needs to warm up when you're full of adrenaline from getting lost and running down from the car park anyway?

Perhaps it's a theme that I carry with me for every event I do, but I wasn't bothered about time. I was focusing on running the entire distance and not letting myself walk when my head got tired. There was quite a lot of support from the local people during the route, which was lovely. It was quite a varied route, and I felt like I'd seen everywhere in Yeovil in one go. It wasn't the easiest route either as there were quite a few inclines, including the famous Hendford Hill (which has its own timing system so that the fastest can be crowned King/Queen of the Hill). I definitely wasn't Queen of the Hill, but I ran the whole way up and felt pretty strong.

This was my first event without headphones and I had been a little worried that I wouldn't get through the event without music, but it turned out not to be an issue. I hadn't once stopped to walk and I felt like I could just keep going. I kept losing track of the mile markers to the point where on the final mile I thought I had over three miles to go so started to mess around a bit – running backwards up the hill and daft stuff like that (no idea why I did that, it's not something I'd normally do). Suddenly I realised the finish line was just around the corner and I'd been wasting minutes messing around on the final approach. I crossed the finish line at two hours and thirty-one minutes, a couple of minutes faster than the last half marathon and while I was pleased that I had made it through without walking, I was also annoyed with myself for missing the opportunity to really run the last mile well and finish under two and a half hours. This was probably the first time I ever felt annoyed about my time. Of course, as soon as I saw my friend she handed me a huge slice of cake and that instantly took my mind off it!

A week before the London Marathon I exceeded my fundraising target of £1800 and was now at £1925, and hoping to make it over £2000 by the big day. I was really working hard to raise the money and get myself ready. I was still following my training plan, which was just short runs at this point. And I was just running outdoors now, unless some treadmill work was beneficial for other reasons (like not wanting to run in the rain – I'm not a wimp, I like a run in the rain, but we had some heavy downpours and since the runs weren't all that long it made sense to hop on the treadmill instead). I was trying to eat really well and healthily

– trying to see the food as fuel (not my strong point!).

The final week of the training plan would end with the marathon itself, with the day before being a rest day, so once I got my final training run completed on the Friday I reflected on the accomplishment of getting through seventeen weeks of marathon training. I'd followed the training plan as closely as was feasible for me. I had my bad weeks, of course. Two long runs got cut short for various reasons and the really long runs were more difficult that I'd expected. I'd had my great weeks too, particularly the Llanelli and Yeovil events and my twenty-two-mile training run. I'd had thoughts about giving up, that there was no way I could complete it, that it was just another thing I was going to fail at, and feeling stupid for even trying. But none of those thoughts mattered now because I'd done it. I had completed seventeen weeks of training for the London Marathon and I had exceeded my fundraising target. Now all I had to do was run the marathon itself. No biggie. I was feeling good – and strong – and I was batting those dark clouds out of sight.

Chapter Ten
Finding strength

As the London weekend approached I was on a high. I'd done absolutely everything I could, other than run the marathon itself. On the coach journey to London Victoria, I was a bag of nerves. Something about actually going to London made the 26.2 miles seem very real and not just a distant thing that was going to happen at some point. My mum and sister had decided to accompany me to London for the weekend and I was grateful for the support. We arrived at Victoria Coach Station just before lunchtime on the Saturday and after a quick coffee, we went straight to the Excel Centre to the marathon expo to register and collect my race number and timing chip. As we were travelling down the day before the event, I didn't have much time to register, so it was so important to get that sorted even before finding our hotel.

After registering, I didn't spend long at the expo. I'm not sure why but I seemed to race through the whole thing and not look at anything on any of the stalls. Probably a good thing, I can imagine it's quite easy to spend a lot of money on the shiny running gear. My purpose was to quickly visit The Children's

Trust stall to say hello to the volunteers and then we were going to head back to Victoria to check in at our hotel, which we'd picked because it was just a short walk from the marathon finish and the coach station. I figured being close to the end would be more helpful than close to the start.

On the morning of the marathon we got up early, ate a quick breakfast and headed to Greenwich. I was really nervous now. I had forced my mum and sister to hurry up with their breakfast (much to my sister's annoyance) because I was so worried about turning up late and not being able to take part. Seeing all the other runners with their race numbers pinned to their tops on the journey there, and their nervous faces, made me feel like I was part of something wider than just myself. The underground/DLR journey to Greenwich was hassle free, and I was glad of it, as it seemed to provide me a little mental preparation time. My mum was getting nervous for me now. She was scanning the faces of the other supporters and registering the nerves emanating from their eyes when they were talking to the runners they were there to support. She made me promise that if I wasn't feeling well I would drop out. I said I would but inside I knew I wouldn't need to. Once we arrived at Greenwich, there were so many other runners and supporters around that it was easy enough to find the start. I was at the red start so just followed the crowd to the starting area. I said goodbye to my mum and sister just outside the entrance to the red start and they headed off into the streets to find a good place to watch and cheer the runners.

After I dropped my bag off at the truck, I spent all my time queuing for the portaloos. That's all I did. I didn't have time for several nervous wees but I think I queued up twice before running over to my starting pen just before we started the slow walk to the start line. It was good to chat to other runners during this time. I think everyone felt exactly the same – delighted and terrified. I was in starting pen number six, so reasonably near to the back but not right at the back where I'd usually choose to start. My start time was ten o'clock but as it took so long to make the painfully slow march to the start line from our pen (cue jokes of 'Oh I think I can handle this if we stick to this pace!'), I didn't actually cross the starting line until about quarter past ten, so we really were at a snail's pace.

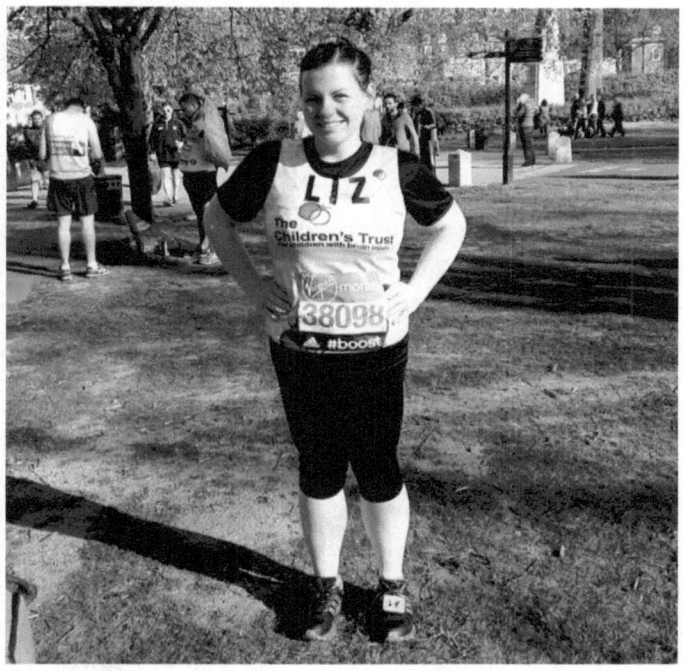

When I could finally see the starting line I had a momentary panic internally but started increasing my pace and ran across it. I started off well and kept my pace slow. It was quite a nice day – warm and sunny, and immediately I was boiling hot, so was sipping water constantly. For the first few miles I think I was in a bit of a daze, sort of in awe and in denial of what I was doing. I was looking around at the people in costume, the people in charity vests like mine but in all different colours to represent the individual charities, and I really felt part of something wonderful. Every runner that day had a story to tell. How many of them were, like me, trying to turn pain into positivity? I choked back tears at certain points because it was just so overwhelming. I was keeping up a steady and manageable pace, one I would have been able to maintain for the full 26.2 miles.

I saw my mum and sister cheering me on from one of the Greenwich streets, so that was fantastic. I really didn't expect to manage to see them given the immense number of runners and supporters, but I did and that meant everything. All was well and I felt strong for the first six-ish miles. And then something happened. I did something awkward to my right foot while running and had pain from my toes around to my ankle, but the worst pain was around the little toe. I ran through the pain for ages, trying to ignore it but it wasn't easing. I stopped twice to take my shoe off but I realised there was nothing I could do except keep going. If I was going to drop out because of this then I would be limping off at less than the halfway point, and that certainly wasn't going to happen. My pace slowed and I had to run/walk/limp, but I kept going. The thing is, I don't really remember actually doing whatever I did, just the pain that occurred. A bit of backstory – I have out-turning feet and spent my childhood in adapted shoes, after an accident as a toddler, so I have to be careful with how I walk/run in general. In day-to-day life I am most comfortable wearing Dr Martens as they provide a lot of support and stop my feet/ankles from randomly turning outwards and making me almost fall, but I'd been lucky to not experience much of this issue while running previously. I can only assume that's what happened as in totally honesty a lot of it was a blur. But I was not going to let this injury stop me from completing the marathon; even if I had to crawl to the finish line, I would do it. No pain was going to stop me. After the euphoria of running over Tower Bridge, and passing the halfway mark, it really started to become tough, but the charity cheering points and the crowds watching were wonderful and kept my spirits up.

In a normal scantily supported event, I might well have dropped out, as I'm pretty sure my head would have won the battle. But, I must say, the spectators were absolutely amazing. Absolutely wonderful. I can't tell you how many times they lifted me when I was ready to give up. Several times someone would centre in on me and get me going again. 'Liz, Liz! If you start running again now, we'll give you the biggest cheer ever!' And off I'd go again. I want to thank those people so much because I wouldn't have got through it without them. I know not everyone enjoys the support along the route, as they prefer to get into their own little running world and ignore everything outside of them, but I relished that support. The crowd figuratively carries some of the runners through the miles and I was most definitely one of them. I did my fair share of high fiving people and tried to interact with the crowds. They were giving to me and I felt I needed to give back in some way. I did some daft dancing at one point when *Insomnia* by Faithless was blasting out of someone's stereo. The atmosphere was immense.

Every time I felt my faith wavering, I told myself to visualise the finish line and see myself crossing it. I told myself to think of the children. I thought particularly of my friend's child who had suffered brain damage as the result of an asthma attack causing a cardiac arrest. I had moments like these frequently, feeling utterly overwhelmed with emotion and thinking of the marathons these children and their carers had to complete every day of their lives. I felt the wider significance of what I was doing. This wasn't just turning my pain into positivity, it was bigger than that. The £2065 I had now raised was going to provide help for others. It was going to provide some positivity for them too. I felt the selfishness of dwelling on my own pain as well. I had evoked the same feelings of struggle I'd experienced during the Cardiff Half, the previous year. It would have been lovely to breeze through the marathon, but clearly I still had things to learn about myself and that was the time. I had more to learn about never giving up. I needed to access strength I didn't know I had. I needed to learn what it really meant to just keep going.

Despite the wonderfulness of the crowd and the atmosphere, the route itself was harder than I expected – even without a dodgy foot it would have been tough. 26.2 miles is a long way and you only start to appreciate just how far it is once you're in the teen miles. I found that the numbers started getting to me. I would forget what the last number was and convince myself I was further forward or further behind than I really was. And then I would either be relieved or gutted when I finally noticed the next mile marker. Marathons are psychologically as well as physically tough, but the crowd lift you, the other runners support you, the scenery and costumes keep you interested and it really is amazing. There were funny little things along the route which I just loved – the sideways showers for one. I ran through every single one I saw. It was welcome relief on a warm day. At one point a priest flung holy water over the runners. He seemed to have his whole congregation out supporting everyone.

Often during an event when you're struggling you'll meet someone else who is also struggling and you'll provide each other the motivation to keep going without even trying. At Canary Wharf I bumped into my cousin's friend and we had a chat (all my cousin had said to me was 'look out for a woman wearing a Welsh flag cowboy hat' but of the forty thousand runners I never expected to actually see her). Just proves that when you need help, it'll find you.

Nearing the end, at mile twenty-five, I broke down in tears. It was a culmination of things, prompted by a young man running near me who was crying. I wondered what had caused his tears, was it the pain of the miles or something more? What was his reason for running today? The sight of him in tears set me off and everything poured out quickly. I cried for everything from our treatment, all the years of infertility and loss, to the hope and dedication that this marathon represented, and even for how my body ached from the event itself. During the last three miles the crowd seemed to be cheering extra hard for us all, probably because our faces were now weary and a lot of people (myself included) were running/walking through tiredness. I kept going, feeling myself being pulled towards the finish line. I turned the corner, almost at the end, and saw Buckingham Palace ahead. I was almost there. I had almost completed the London Marathon.

When I finally ran through the final six hundred metres and across the finish line on The Mall, I felt this huge burst of excitement rush through my body. There were no more miles left to run. I had done it. I had run a marathon. The London Marathon. I raised my hands up in the air as I crossed the line, my hands formed into fists, punching the air above me. When I approached the lady who was poised ready to put my medal over my head, I held out my hand to high five her, she joined in and then congratulated me. I looked down at my medal and felt emotional. If anyone had told me in the past that I would have my own London Marathon medal placed around my neck, I would have thought they were insane. I had actually run a marathon and I was so proud – yes it had taken me six hours and fifteen minutes to do it (seventy-five minutes longer than planned), but I didn't care for one moment. It was one of the best things I had ever done. Every moment of pain, every moment of doubt, every moment of the training plan, had all been worth it. I had achieved what I had set out to do, for the first time in as long as I could remember.

Walking at a slow pace was welcome and almost relaxing, so the walk to find my family really helped my tense muscles and sore foot. I had little idea of where I was going, and when I rang my mum to find out where they were, I told them I was in a completely different place than I was, because I was so overwhelmed and I didn't know what I was saying. Luckily I walked straight towards them without even realising. They'd had a fantastic day as spectators (managed to see Mo Farah and the rest of the elite up close) and they were happy that I had arrived at the end in one piece!

Unfortunately, I didn't make it to the charity's after party (which I was upset about), as I just wanted to get back to the hotel to rest my foot. Not that I got any rest, however. I found that once I lay down my muscles just screamed at me. I managed to cheer on a few finishers on the way back, who were almost at the end. I could see the determination and relief in their eyes; they were almost there. They had made it through 26.2 miles. It was wonderful to see. All I achieved that evening (aside from showering as soon as we got back to the hotel – perhaps the best shower ever) was to go across the road for a meal in the pub. I kept looking at my medal with alternating disbelief and pride.

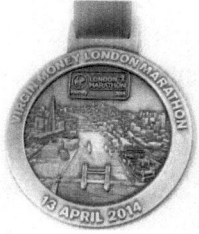 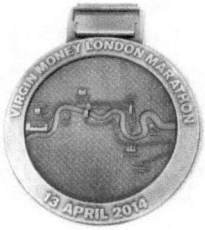

The next morning, the breakfast room was filled with runners and their families, so we all shared our stories of the event. There was still a lovely positive atmosphere and aside from the one poor woman who was unable to get out of her bed (according to her sister) everyone was still in high spirits. We were heading home after breakfast, so I wore my finishers t-shirt as we walked from our hotel to the coach station and people continued to congratulate me. One man told me that he had run the marathon the previous year but 'couldn't walk for three bloody days' after, so I thought I was doing pretty well.

I hadn't realised how much I'd needed to learn about myself and about life. Sometimes a struggle is a learning opportunity, and in that marathon I'd learnt so much. Not just from my own personal experience but from the other runners and from the spectators. I'd appreciated the generosity of the support from the crowds, I'd seen the determination, the pain, and the jubilation on the faces of the other runners, and I'd seen myself succeed in a way I couldn't have predicted. Being obese for the majority of my life had meant that the idea of even running down the road was laughable, but I'd now learnt that a new way of living was possible. I'd lost the weight I never thought I'd be able to lose. I'd gained fitness that I never expected to gain. And now I'd run a marathon which previously would only have been possible in my wildest dreams. Nothing would take away the dashed desire to have my own child, but there was so much else I was learning. If you really set your mind to something, you could achieve it. It just may not look the way you thought it would. But that's the humour of life, always a surprise.

A few thoughts kept running through my head:
Trust yourself. Believe in yourself. Learn to love yourself.

CHAPTER ELEVEN
You must be crazy

I got knocked off my London high by a nasty virus. On reflection, I'd shown initial signs of the virus the day before the marathon but I was too preoccupied to be really aware of them. Sometimes I wonder if hurting my foot was divine intervention and was a way of making myself take it easy during the event because my body knew it was in the beginning stages of fighting a cold. Who knows? But it made me take an extended rest period, which was very much required. It offered me a time to reflect as well. After I was back to normal health, I found myself looking for what I could do next to keep my spirits high and my thoughts positive. I had the Wales Marathon planned but that was a couple of months away. I was still updating my blog, still focused on exercise, still working, still volunteering, still sharing my story. So I just kept going.

I pondered the words that had stuck with me after finishing the marathon. Those words were highlighting things in my life and things I saw around me. As I was becoming more and more involved with the fitness/diet world I was starting to find certain things troubling. One thing that I found alarming was how people never seemed to be happy or satisfied with themselves. I'd seen myself experience some of that with the burgeoning BMI obsession, which luckily I got under control. But it saddened me that people (often myself included) seemed to be at war with their bodies, rather than at peace. People always seemed to have something about their body or themselves that they absolutely hated. One of the things that was becoming more and more clear to me was that I needed to learn to love myself. I needed to love my body, even the parts that didn't look or work exactly as I wanted them to. I needed to even love my reproductive system, even though I felt like it had constantly let me down. It is no easy feat so try and change your mind on deeply ingrained personal ideologies, however. No matter how thin I became, I would still have loose skin on my stomach, a common occurrence with weight loss. No matter how healthy or fit I became, my PCOS symptoms would still be there, maybe lessened, but a distinct lack of a pregnancy despite never using contraception would prove my inability to conceive month after month. My narrow hips and broad shoulders gave me a 'manly' figure according to body shape information online. And while it was the easy option to remain at war with these 'problems', it wasn't solving anything and ultimately kept causing pain.

I didn't want to go through each day of my life at war with my own body. I made the decision to refuse to. The thing was, because I'd spent most of my life obese then lost weight, the old insecurities didn't just dissipate, they'd stuck around, and sometimes they'd intensified, even taking on new forms. I'd never be thin enough, fit enough, or pretty enough. But I was done with that. I wanted to let it go. I didn't want to walk around caring what other people thought of me or my body. I ran and worked out because I loved my body and wanted to take care of it, not to punish myself. It saddened me that often people couldn't see just how awesome our bodies really are. We are all beautiful. We are all amazing. But for some reason we allow current societal standards of beauty or ill health to sabotage our relationship with ourselves. I got on the road to self-acceptance and did my best to never look back.

I was now in a place where I was no longer annoyed that God or the universe had let me down and stripped me of my dreams. I had rebuilt my faith brick by brick in the same way I had rebuilt my life, and despite the normal doubts and confusion that was common in my life, I really felt like I was in some way back on track. Of course, I would be lying if I didn't admit that had I been offered the chance of having my own child, I would have swapped everything I had for it wholeheartedly, but getting pregnant no longer dominated my waking thoughts in quite the same way. 'Believe in yourself' was becoming my mantra and I would remind myself of it whenever I was feeling low. And I did still have my low moments. I hadn't run them away entirely.

My next running event was the Beast of Bryn – there were two versions, a 15-mile route or a 6.8-mile route, both going up through the mountains. I had registered for the 15-mile version, thinking it would be a good training run for the next marathon and really it would have been, but something on the day wasn't right at all. It was a warm day and I just wasn't feeling it. This was the first time where I knew I wasn't going to be able to finish the race. I met some ladies who were swapping to the shorter route and I did the same. It was that or suffer a DNF (did not finish) and I wanted to at least accomplish something that day, even if it was only 6.8 miles. That morning I had struggled to get myself out of the house to even drive to the event, so it wasn't as if my motivation was never ending. I had off days when my heart wasn't in it. I had days when I wanted to give up.

Though it was an extremely challenging trail run, the views were just divine. During the massive hill climbs I walked with the ladies I had met at the start. It was nice to feel social, as I had so far only run events by myself. All 'failures' are a learning opportunity and I realised immediately what I needed to learn that day – it's okay to take it easy. Just like that cold forced me into an extended rest period after the marathon, I was understanding more about the necessity of rest and how being left alone with my thoughts wasn't as bad as it previously had been. Swapping the distances didn't mean I'd messed up or failed anything, it just meant that on that day I had listened to how I felt and completed the shorter route instead, and that was okay. I had more of an awareness now of seeing the bigger picture. When I crossed the finish line of the 6.8-mile route, I had the same satisfaction as I always did. It really is the taking part that counts. It's the effort that matters. It reiterated what I had already realised, that when things don't go to plan perhaps we are just being offered the chance to learn, either about ourselves or about life, and we just have to be open to seeing it.

While working on my training plan leading up to the Wales Marathon, I had made the decision to raise money for my friend's son who had been present in my thoughts during the London Marathon. I was going to do a 10k event on the first Sunday, the marathon on the middle Sunday and then finish with a half marathon the Sunday after. A summer challenge. So I was doing my best to raise what I could. I'd done a lot of fundraising over the past year but people still gave generously. I was chugging along with my marathon training plan, although it was going very differently this time. My longest training run was sixteen miles and I felt a lot more laid back. I suppose I was more secure in my own personal knowledge that I could complete a marathon, so I simply stressed less. I was also doing more cross training, so I was building up more strength and fitness doing circuit and weight training.

A few weeks before the 10k I was walking around Tenby in West Wales (coincidentally the same town in which the marathon was due to take place) with my husband, and I saw a crystal shop with a sign in the window offering card readings. My husband (not a partaker in this sort of thing but nevertheless understood my interest) suggested that I have a reading. So I booked a time with the lady and went back later for my card reading. My husband sat in on the reading but it was me alone that was choosing the cards and conversing with the reader.

I was in two minds about doing it because I'd wasted my time with those online pregnancy readings years ago and I'd been left with false hope after my two in person readings the previous year, but something about it felt right, so I was receptive. The lady doing the reading was down to earth and funny, she wasn't at all who you'd expect to be giving readings in a crystal shop. She definitely did not fit the stereotype. And the shop itself was light and bright, not at all like what you'd probably see on an old film with a dark and dingy incense-filled back room. This put me at ease as well. I don't remember how many cards I picked or what they were, but there were a lot of things she seemed to understand and she gave us advice on some forthcoming situations. But then she mentioned a baby. A baby was coming to us next year, in the spring. I asked her if she was referring to a natural pregnancy or via fertility treatment (not that we had anything planned but I had found myself googling fertility clinics a couple of times over the previous few weeks). She retrieved a crystal on a silver chain from a velvet purse and dowsed the question. The answer that came to her was 'leave it to God'.

When the reading was coming to its natural end she asked me

to pick one card from a different deck for a final message. The card was 'Believe in Yourself'. I looked at her and for that one moment everything seemed to be right, perfect as it was. I thanked her and we left. This was my husband's first experience of a reading and it had been quite interesting for him. We discarded her message about a baby almost instantly, we both knew not to dwell on any messages about children. We didn't need any false hope. So we largely forgot what she said and I just took the final message away with me.

That parting message stayed with me and helped me through the final weeks before the three events. Of course, I was excited to do them but I was also anxious. It was a reasonably hot summer and I'd read scare stories about people passing out during summer marathons. Typical pre-marathon thoughts when the ego tries to take over. I may not have run the distances in training that I did in my first marathon training but due to the diversity of cross training in general I was feeling all round stronger. I'd managed to raise £260, which was gratefully received by the trust for my friend's son.

Despite my strong attempts to move on from the idea of any further fertility treatment, I'd had a few shaky moments where I had contacted a couple of private fertility clinics to enquire about egg sharing (which could provide heavily discounted treatment if accepted). This would mean that I would donate some of the retrieved eggs to another woman at the same time as having treatment for myself. I couldn't quite find the right information as to whether we would qualify, considering I hadn't ever been a massive responder to the drugs and the last cycle had been a disaster. The replies I received all told me that they'd need to see my notes and it would be best to come in for a proper consultation.

General enquiries were one thing, but I didn't want to go in to see anyone, so nothing went any further than those initial enquiries. My husband and I both knew that we didn't want to go back into the IVF bubble. Not so soon, anyway. And I knew deep down that adoption would be our next step, not more treatment. I had made such progress and it felt like more treatment really would be a backwards step. So I filed the idea away, and my husband and I decided to revisit it in the future if the urge returned, but for now it wasn't right for us.

I had five running events planned for the rest of the year: Llanelli 10k, Wales Marathon, Swansea Half Marathon, Bristol Half Marathon and then ending with the Cardiff Half Marathon in October. Running and events had now become my hobby, something I just enjoyed doing. At this point I was just interested in plodding along rather than pushing myself to achieve faster times. I figured I had plenty of time to work on faster times in the years to come. I was feeling a bit overwhelmed though, and I was slowly trying to detangle myself from the myriad of things I'd volunteered for, my job, plus the work I was doing outside of work, because I really had spread myself too thin.

We had shared our infertility story with a couple of news publications and a magazine, as an infertility charity had asked us if we would like to be involved. While we weren't terribly keen on getting too heavily involved in that sort of thing, we felt that if sharing our experiences helped someone else then it would be worth it. Seeing our story on news websites or in print was a bit odd though. I never ever read the comments. One particular time involved a full photoshoot to accompany the article. A photographer and a makeup artist/hairdresser turned up at my house and I was completely thrown by this. It wasn't something I was used to. The magazine editors had had specific ideas about the photoshoot and I point blank refused most of them. There was no way I was going to stand outside primary school gates or in a children's park, looking morose. I felt that that would have made a mockery of my situation and other people who were also suffering. As it was, standing out in public having my photo taken by a professional photographer felt strange enough, I didn't want to feel like an idiot outside some random school gates. I was willing to share my story but not in a way that made me uncomfortable.

The first event of the summer challenge was the Llanelli 10k. It was nice to return to the route but I had mixed feelings when thinking back to the previous year's event. This was the first time I was running with anyone I knew (my husband – his very first event – and a friend from work) and I appreciated the company. It was a sunny day and the heat seemed to be radiating upwards from the tarmac of the coastal path, so it seemed like a different experience from the previous year. Weather aside, I felt like an entirely different person to who I'd been during the event last year. During that event I was stuck between the heartbreak of the first IVF cycle and the hope of the second, I still very much believed that the second cycle would be successful for us, and I'd run with a sort of carefree hope. Hope that had dissolved the moment I'd received that phone call from the embryologist.

Now I was running the same route, and I couldn't help but think about all that had occurred, but I felt different. I had more battle scars but I felt like a more evolved person somehow, like I had faced a crippling fear and come through the other side. It was a thought provoking 6.2 miles. And it was nice to have people with me for once. Running with them was a reminder to snap back to the present and not live in my thoughts of the past. I finished with a slower time than the previous year but that wasn't relevant to me, I was one third of the way through my challenge and had the marathon to think of the next weekend, so this was no time for a PB (personal best). Crossing the finish line of each event was my goal.

The next Sunday came around quickly and once again it was obvious that I had signed up for an event with no idea of the terrain. In the case of the Wales Marathon, I had heard a couple of people say it 'had some hills' but that was as much as I knew about the route. A friend of mine was also running the marathon (the same friend who inspired me by running the London Marathon in 2012), but as he was considerably faster than me, we wouldn't be starting together and I wouldn't see him on the route either. The marathon was part of the Long Course Weekend, which included swimming on the Friday, cycling on the Saturday and then running on the Sunday. The marathon alone was challenge enough for me. The route started and ended in Tenby, a pretty coastal town in West Wales, so before registering and finding some last minute toilets, we sat on some benches near the start and looked out to sea. It didn't seem to be too hot, so my fears of passing out in the sun were unfounded. I had a lot of support that day from friends and family who were all there to watch the event.

Not long after we got started I realised that this was going to be a really challenging experience. It was very steep in places, but I was happy enough going along at my own pace. I was in a good mood so I was stopping to talk to the marshals at the water stands and taking in the sights around me. I assured myself that all these hills must just be in the first half, not the whole way though, surely? Then I overheard someone say that the second half was even worse. Uh-oh, I was starting to panic a little now. Although judging by my estimated time, I was still on course to finish between five and five and a half hours, so despite numerous walking breaks, as long as I kept going, I was golden. The volunteers were really friendly and encouraging, so

I felt uplifted by that. This was a different type of marathon altogether from London. Due to the types of roads, there were few supporters (other than in the towns) so it was better to go into your own little world.

When the hills just kept coming, I was half amused and half furious. But at no point did I consider giving up, and the distance didn't bother me in the same way it had done in London. Okay, I hadn't injured myself this time, so I had that on my side, but once I got to halfway, I just knew I would make it all the way to the end. Instead of looking at the numbers going up and getting overwhelmed by them, I reversed it and saw it as a countdown. I was very close to the back so I was only ever running with a couple of runners either in front or behind me. But I never felt totally alone as I had done in that twenty-mile event in Llanelli. I kept running/walking, becoming more and more aware that I was now going to finish around the six hour mark, but all I wanted to do was finish. Completing this challenging route was enough for me.

I honestly don't remember dwelling significantly during this event, perhaps the words 'believe in yourself' had really taken hold and I knew that I would get to the end, come what may. I had fleeting thoughts about all the ways in which I felt I'd failed over the years, but every time I turned a corner and saw another hill, I almost laughed about it. It was almost like life itself. Whenever I thought things were going smoothly, I'd turn a corner and there'd be another challenge staring me in the face. Quite near the end I completely lost track of the miles and the route, so it was almost a surprise to me when I reached the top of the hill, turned right and saw the finishing line ahead. I sprinted like crazy when I saw it. And because I was one of the last ones back I was alone running down the red carpet and alone running under the finish line when I crossed it at around six hours and five minutes. The streets were lined with people all cheering for me and I heard them call my name out over the loud speaker to encourage me to the end. I swear it felt like I had won that race, and my race photos really illustrate that. Just me, not just winning my own personal marathon but winning my own personal battle as well. I'll never forget how I felt in that moment. Purely elated.

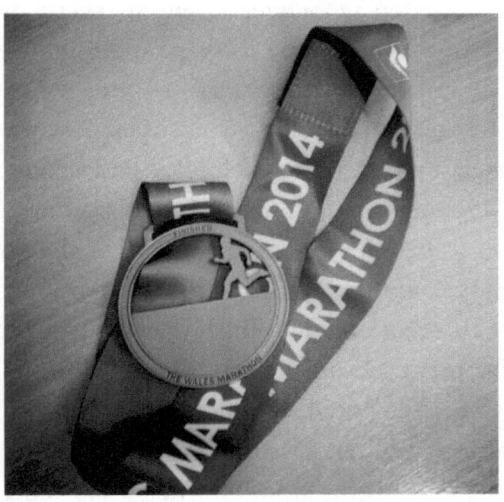

The final event of the challenge was the inaugural Swansea Half Marathon, the next Sunday. It was a warm, sunny day and while I had no ill effects from the previous weekend's marathon, I knew it was going to be another slow event for me. I suppose I just didn't have the inclination after doing so many events in a short space of time to push myself. I think I was still on a high from the marathon as well, so I was off with a good steady (albeit slow) pace and my mind was calm. I no longer worried about whether or not I would reach the finish line during these events – I knew I could. I had done a lot of my marathon training along the seafront in Swansea, so running the half marathon that day along a route I was familiar with gave me a really nice feeling.

When I'd been training I'd been full of doubt and fear, but here I was, already having done the two marathons, just chugging along, almost blissfully, looking out to sea, full of gratitude for the strength in my legs to carry me forward. The water seemed to be a sparkling crystal blue that day, calm and peaceful. I tried to carry that peaceful vision with me. I was happy to see spectators along the route cheering everyone and I did my best to look excited and animated whenever I saw an event photographer (this is a very hit or miss thing to do, sometimes the photos are good, sometimes just hilariously awful). Once the route diverted away from the seafront I really wasn't sure where we were going, so for the last couple of miles I felt like I had accidentally veered off course and was just running around confused. For some reason I tend to lose my orientation towards the end of events and this was yet another where the end came as a complete shock to me. But crossing that finish line was just a lovely feeling of accomplishment. I'd finished the summer running challenge, raised all the money I could, and developed a place for myself to foster whatever happiness I could find. The difference between my mental state at events now to when I started running was considerable. Once filled with an inescapable feeling of just not being good enough, I was now filled with a calm knowingness and a belief in myself.

The thing with life is that happiness and sadness seem to approach in waves. Sometimes you're riding high and sometimes you're being dragged under the waves, trying not to drown. I had really worked hard to rebuild my life after it all crashed down. I'd found ways of feeling peaceful and happy and strong, but that didn't mean that I had entirely released myself from the weights that lurked beneath the surface. I'd cut away a lot of my expectations but every now and then one would tug at my ankle and threaten to flood everything. This would primarily hit me when I was at work, alone. I was tremendously unfulfilled in my job, and so when I'd get frustrated by the mundane nature of the task at hand it would allow my mind to focus on all the things I didn't have and all the ways in which I had failed and was unhappy. I would think about all the people who fell pregnant without trying that didn't even want to be pregnant, I would think about the people that were seemingly just handed whatever it was they wanted on a plate with no effort needed, and I felt bitter. I would struggle to keep myself from breaking down as I felt like there was little point to my life. I remember staring blankly at the computer screen in a silent office, nothing but the hum of activity downstairs to be heard, and I would wonder exactly what the point of life was. I would think about the many, many successful people who had achieved so many wonderful things but when they were asked what their best achievement was, they'd all say their children. Was this something they felt obligated to say? Or was their love for their children simply greater than all other achievements? No matter what I achieved, would the ache in my heart still be there?

The wish to have a baby can lie dormant, but I don't think it ever truly leaves you. You can find happiness and fulfilment in other ways, of course, and I do mean genuine happiness, but it's a wound that never completely heals. It's as if it's been stitched up incompetently and at risk of tearing open at a moment you cannot predict.

Nevertheless, I had done all I could in a reasonably short time to accept that I wouldn't have my own children through my own pregnancy and tried to release the need or expectation for it to happen miraculously. And the peace from this decision would be present in waves, just like the pain. Just like the dark clouds, sometimes they were straight in front of me, and sometimes they were lurking at the sides. When I thought back over the

Little Something

rollercoaster of the last few years I was amazed. I could see how I'd evolved, how my world had changed, but there was still that space in my heart for a child, and I wasn't sure if we were ready or not, but I thought it might be time to consider adoption.

CHAPTER TWELVE
Why don't you just adopt?

As the autumn began and we were approaching a full year since our final IVF cycle had ended so abruptly, we relocated about an hour's drive away. This move was a big, positive step for us. It would force me to change jobs, it would mean my husband had a considerably shorter commute and it would be a chance to shed the weight that the old house contained. We'd seen some dark moments in that house, so leaving it behind was freeing.

Moving house is all-consuming, so all running and other activities had taken a back seat to packing, and then unpacking, and settling into our new house and area. We were now living in a newly built house which wasn't bogged down by old energy, and this move was a step forward in creating a different life for ourselves. We no longer lived up in the mountains but down by the sea, with the cleansing sea air to reinvigorate us. I had signed up for a fitness course and was working on that, and looking for new jobs, so it seemed like we were in a better place to consider adoption. We needed at least a full year to really grieve our loss, and now we were getting ready to learn about the process of adoption, but aside from doing research online, we weren't quite ready to contact any adoption agencies just yet. I was finding myself less preoccupied by other people's pregnancy or birth announcements. They still evoked certain feelings but I didn't find them quite so overwhelming. My sister-in-law was pregnant with our niece and despite the initial kicks to the gut which were just jealousy surfacing, I was really excited to become an aunt and for the wider family to grow.

It wasn't long before the Cardiff Half Marathon had rolled around again. Sadly, I'd had to miss the Bristol Half Marathon due to a virus, so I was keen to get back to health so that I could complete the Cardiff Half. It was more symbolic than anything. I had taken part the previous year battered and broken and now I was more complete and stronger. I had also decided that I would do the London Marathon again, the next year. So was looking forward to attending that event as a stronger person as well. This time the Cardiff Half felt different. It felt fun. It was such a contrast to the year before. I almost fell over about a mile in, but I laughed it off and kept going.

The route was almost identical, so I could remember how I felt at the different points a year ago. It's a strange thing, but repeating events year after year makes you compare to the previous years. In some ways, it made me wonder why I had done the event the previous year. My body wasn't okay and neither was my mind, but I'd made the decision to do it, and it was a gesture, a symbol. A promise that I was making myself.

I wasn't really aware of it entirely at the time but taking part was me telling myself that I believed in myself, believed in my life and knew that I could get through anything. I learnt a lesson that sticks with me to this day – just keep going. Looking back, it felt like I had squished weeks of therapy into those three hours and thirteen minutes. It was a healing experience and it was what I needed to do to push myself forward. So now I was running it again, and it wasn't my fastest half marathon but it wasn't anywhere near my slowest, either. Maybe thirty-five minutes faster than the previous year. I remember looking around and just taking in my surroundings, I knew that this event was finishing off a year which had been, in many ways, the hardest one of my life. Sure, the treatment had ended, so I hadn't had that to deal with over the past year, but I'd had to grieve and to rebuild, and that really was momentous. I felt like I had learnt so much about myself, so when I crossed the finish line that day I felt emotional because I really had come full circle.

Later that month I turned thirty-one. I was driving home from work on my birthday and had a distinct moment of clarity flood my mind out of nowhere. I thought about all I'd achieved with the weight loss and the running and I suddenly realised that if I went back in time and told my previous self what I was going to do I would have said it was a dream come true, miraculous. I never really thought I would be able to do anything like that. But I had. So that day, on my thirty-first birthday, I wrote a blog post about how I was grateful for my life and was looking forward to more of my dreams coming true. I acknowledged that at thirty-one I was healthier than I'd been at twenty-one or even at eleven. Of course, another thought ran through my head – I was now thirty-one; I was twenty-four when I stopped taking the mini pill. Since I was well-informed that fertility declined with age, it was less likely that I would become naturally pregnant now than I would have at twenty-four, surely? It seemed like the door was well and truly closed on that part of my life. Adoption or a childless/childfree life was lying ahead of us, we just didn't know which.

After my birthday, things seemed to change in quick succession. I gave notice at work as I'd found a new job, then I did the attendance part of my fitness trainer course. While I had been looking forward to doing this course, it became a source of anxiety. I kept thinking I wasn't fit, thin or good enough to do it, which was just my ego giving me a hard time. That week was actually quite refreshing as it shook up my whole routine. It was nice spending a week doing something totally different to my day-to-day job.

At the start of December I started my new job. It wasn't my dream job but it was a different job, and that's what I needed, change. At that time it was very important to us to plan the coming year. I wanted to focus on my personal development and growth, and my husband had his own difficulties to overcome. By the end of December I had registered for seven events for 2015, including two marathons, and we tried to make a couple of the events into weekends away so that we would get some time together as well.

I was fundraising for another children's charity (MACS) for the London Marathon and had instigated a virtual run to raise funds for the charity. I was feeling pretty focused on the year ahead and looking forward to it. Of course, Christmas can be a trying time and I had more than one moment of bitterness and sadness, which I unloaded on my husband and heavily pregnant sister-in-law, but overall I was doing well. As the new year rolled in, I felt all the possibilities and opportunities come alive in my mind. I knew it was going to be a good year.

As January began, I often found myself feeling annoyed with myself. Not because I was infertile but because I'd allowed myself to become so wrapped up with being infertile for so many years. In all that time the focus had been on pregnancy and other things had been pushed aside. I hadn't established a career and I just felt like I hadn't done enough with those years.

After thinking back to the previous year and all I'd achieved, I felt like I'd allowed trying to conceive and fertility treatment to rob myself of a career, and other wonderful things that were possible. It was way too easy to condemn myself and say that I wish I'd had a little more perspective at the time and realised that life wasn't all about trying to get pregnant. But that's all too simple to say on reflection.

At the time, wanting to have a baby was my world and even when other things were happening it was an undercurrent, a constant element lurking at the corner of every conversation. From making the decision to stop using contraception to the end of our fertility treatment was over five years. And in all those years I honestly didn't have one meaningful job, and nothing with any career progression. Yes, I'd finished my research degree, but once that was done I felt stale and unsure where to go next. I made a couple of attempts and applied for many, many jobs, but ultimately I wanted to be a mother and that came first to me. I realised that when our second IVF treatment cycle ended, I wasn't just left childless but also careerless, and as a result I struggled to find meaning in what I was doing.

I am sure that's why my hobby of running took such precedence. I have to take responsibility for this. I could have worked towards gaining a meaningful career, but I didn't. Not everyone puts the other aspects of their life on hold while undertaking fertility treatment, but that was the decision I'd made. Truthfully, I didn't believe that anyone would want to hire someone doing fertility treatment, I didn't think anyone would want to hire a failure – because as horrible as it is to admit, infertility made me feel like a failure. And this feeling of failure extended into everything.

During the previous year I had gained back some of the belief that I'd lost and I'd stepped outside of my comfort zone.

Suffering with infertility did not make me a failure, nor does it make anyone else a failure. Not establishing a career by my early thirties also didn't make me a failure, nor does it make anyone else a failure. I'd learnt so much about myself and about life over the years and was glad to have embraced a more positive outlook as a result, even if it was a bit shaky and slipped through my fingers at times. I thought a lot about how people felt when going through infertility, and how the different types of infertility affect people. I suppose for my husband and me, we were on an equal footing as we both had issues which rendered us infertile. I wondered what sort of dynamic occurred when the issues were on one side only. How did they feel? We both blamed ourselves anyway, so was that feeling magnified in different scenarios? And how did people come to terms with unexplained infertility? When there's seemingly nothing wrong on either side, but it just isn't happening? Was it immensely frustrating waiting and waiting for the time to be right? It must have been. I felt that knowing what was wrong and being forced to accept that it wasn't going to happen did force us to let it go. It made us find a way to move on, otherwise we could have stayed in that place and dwelled on it forever.

I became hyperfocused on the awareness of what it was like to be infertile or struggle to conceive. It felt like I could spot it a mile off. I could usher a conversation away from the subject without anyone noticing to spare someone having to deal with their awkward response. I would speak up about the inappropriateness of asking questions in the first place. I tried to become a little voice in the darkness to help people whenever I could. This was why I had decided to share my story – I wanted people to know that they weren't alone.

We'd spoken about adoption a few times by this point, but the time was approaching for us to take a tentative step towards the possibility. Whenever people would ask whether we wanted to adopt, it would come across in a condescending, dismissive manner.

Examples:

1. Have you not thought about adoption then?

2. Why don't you just adopt a baby?

3. Aren't there loads of kids who need homes? Just adopt one.

4. Why haven't you tried to adopt yet?

5. You could get a foreign child – they're crying out for people to do that, aren't they?

6. Can't you just adopt a baby so that we'll have babies at the same time?

Sometimes these comments would drive me slightly crazy and other times I would let them just float away, realising that the people behind the comments just didn't know anything about the process or what kind of emotional toll it took on people. They just saw it in a flippant way and more than likely genuinely believed that it was an easy process.

I'd googled and researched as much as I could but the time had arrived for us to talk to someone about the process, because you can google as much as you like but sometimes the answer to your question just isn't there. I'd contacted a charity adoption agency and the local authority and set up meetings. The first one was with the charity agency. That meeting was relaxed and open – the information and the process were overwhelming but the lady had been so candid and realistic and happy to answer questions that it felt like it might actually be the right thing for us. I'd bought a special tin of expensive biscuits and offered her a selection of drinks, as if that made a huge difference to our chances, which is silly really, as if the decision would be made on our initial meeting alone. The more time we spent talking to her, the more questions arose. Sometimes you don't realise you even have certain questions until discussion prompts them.

One thing (which may seem silly to others) that bothered me was that you didn't necessarily get to name or rename your adopted children. And this bothered me because I'd always liked the idea of naming my children. I communicated this to the lady and she was completely understanding. I envisioned what it might be like to adopt two children (two because we had a small three-bedroom house) and having a ready-made family, something we still yearned for deep down. I knew it would be hard work and taxing but surely worth it in the end? The lady explained the process in its entirety and if we wanted to go forward with the initial application our next step would be to book onto the agency's information course and then potentially an official application would be commenced upon its completion. I was surprised to find out that, in some cases, the process was only around nine months long. The length of a pregnancy could unite an adoptive family.

There seemed to be a lot of reasons why this was the right route for us, but we weren't entirely sure we were ready to embark. The lady encouraged us to speak to the local authority as well as the possibility of a younger child was more likely through them. I wasn't overly fixated on ages, but I will admit that I found the idea of an older child too overwhelming at that point. I think when you've been imagining a baby for so long it takes a while to shift your mindset.

Unfortunately, the experience with the local authority was a complete contrast. Two women turned up and both brought a frost in with them. My questions were unanswered, and they mainly talked at us and didn't want to be interrupted. They discussed sibling sets and when my husband said that four children would be too much to adopt at one go the meeting soured considerably. They didn't seem to understand that this was a nerve-wracking thing for us, and yes, going from no children to four would more than likely have been too much in one go! I got the overwhelming feeling that us having questions at all was a bad thing to them. But who could approach this process without having questions? I can't imagine ever not having questions about something so serious and such a massive commitment.

I think we were both glad to see those two ladies leave because they had set us completely on edge. It was a shame because that meeting really put us off, whereas the meeting with the lady from the other agency had been so encouraging. We were left unsure of what to do. One thing that wasn't a difficult decision was which route to follow when we were ready – the local authority or the charity. We decided on the charity without a second thought and even tentatively booked onto one of their courses a few months away, purely for more information at that point.

For some reason doubts began to set in. Not about adoption specifically, but about the timing. We were finally in a good place as a couple, and individually we were healing, so the thought nagged at the back of both our minds – not now. We didn't tell many people that we were meeting with the adoption agencies, partially because we weren't keen on dealing with the ridiculous comments (fuelled by lack of knowledge and understanding) and partially because we weren't sure if we were ready.

A thought returned to my head from the psychic reading I'd had two years previously – 'you'll have your family at once' – which at the time myself and the medium assumed meant the

IVF treatment leading to twins. But now I was pondering these words all over again… 'at once'… would that be adopting more than one child, siblings probably, at once? I can't say for sure why these words came back to me but they did and I found new meaning in them. It made me wonder what else he had told me that I'd forgotten. I'd already forgotten most of what the lady had told me in the previous year's card reading, so I had little chance of retaining the information from two years ago. But it was obviously still there, hidden away in my mind somewhere, otherwise these words wouldn't have come to me again.

I remember speaking to a friend of a friend who'd adopted a boy and a girl, and I also sought the opinion of a colleague who had been adopted as a baby. I thought the more I understood, the better prepared I would be. But despite everything, the feeling in the pit of my stomach told me that it wasn't the right time. After many discussions we decided that we would shelve the idea for now and discuss it in a year or so. We needed to be 'just a couple' for a while and were still settling into our new surroundings as our own little family.

I think other people found our decision to not have any further fertility treatment and to put an indefinite pause on our interest in adoption confusing. How can you go from wanting a child so much to suddenly not wanting one? People just didn't understand that we hadn't just suddenly stopped wanting one; we had just decided that being a couple and focusing on ourselves was what we needed to do instead. We'd been through such a lot together and in some ways I was amazed that we'd survived it in such good shape. Sadly, not all marriages or relationships survive infertility. We focused more on the things we liked doing, like going out for dinner, going away for the night, running together, just little things. I was no longer questioning whether or not I would be pregnant each month and when my period came it was never a surprise, as I knew it would come. It had been a long time since I had taken a pregnancy test and I was no longer tempted to take any 'just in case'.

It was now early February 2015 and I was half marathon ready again after taking it easy over the festive period. I was on my way down to Brighton to meet up with friends and run the half marathon. My husband couldn't come due to work commitments so he was going to meet me in Cardiff on my way back for us to go out for a meal and have a night away. On the morning of the half marathon it was terrifically cold. The ground by the start was icy. But something about running by the sea and breathing in the salty, fresh, bracing air always felt very cleansing to me, so I ran that race with only thoughts of things that were forthcoming, not the past.

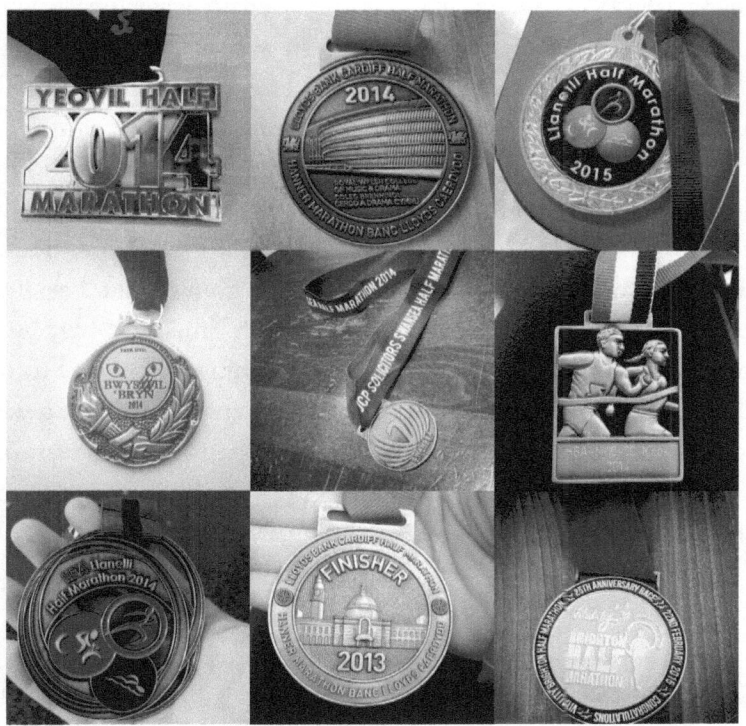

I had even managed to take part in a fitness course for training ante/postnatal women. I had spent an entire weekend talking about and practising training pregnant women and I had got through the entire time without sinking into low mood. Part of me worked extra hard to keep my mood positive, but the other part really was okay. I was pleased with myself because a year before that I would never have got through the course, in fact, even six months before I wouldn't have. But now I was able to attend a course and complete coursework focusing on the one thing I had never been able to achieve, and it didn't cause me to have a breakdown. I'd had a couple of bad moods over the coursework but nothing compared to how I used to feel. This was progress and I had worked hard for it.

Over the years I'd spent a lot of time working out to Jillian Michaels' DVDs in my living room. Before I started running I would see her six days a week, so when she brought her Maximise Your Life tour to the UK I knew I had to go. Luckily at that time I was able to buy a VIP ticket, which meant I got to meet her after the show and have photos taken. I found her show really inspirational and I was feeling really motivated and fired up while watching her speak. When the time came to meet her afterwards I thought through all the things that I wanted to say to her. I knew I wouldn't get much time with her, but I thought I could at least say a couple of things. I wanted to tell her how much meeting her meant to me, what I'd achieved with her help, stuff like that. And then I got in the room, she came up to me and said hello. I said hello in return. We hugged and then I said... nothing. No words came out. I posed for the photos with her and then left. This was a moment that I had been so excited for and yet I had no words to impart. Typical.

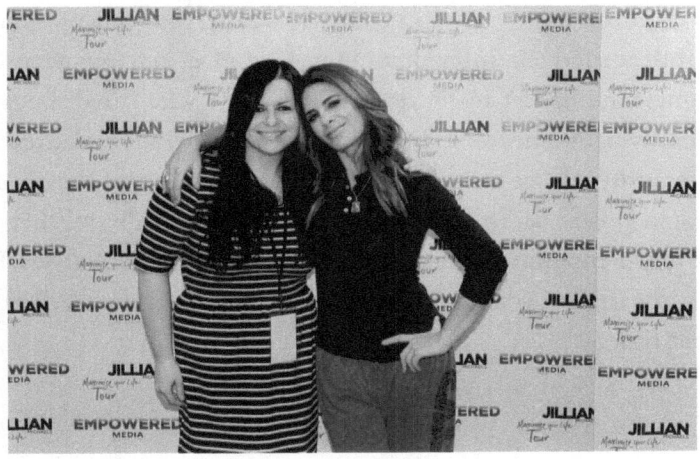

My husband and I had been training together as he was due to run his first half marathon at the beginning of March, the Llanelli Half Marathon. This was his second event after doing the 10k the previous summer. It felt good that he had found some enjoyment (even if it was purely for general fitness) in running, as I liked having a running partner for training and events. We ran that half marathon through the pouring rain (with soaking wet socks) and it felt like something we had achieved together. Afterwards he decided to sign up for a couple of other events as well, so it was clear that he had caught the running bug too. I was deep into marathon training, so it was great to finally have some company.

I half knew and half didn't quite realise the severity, but my husband was battling his own demons. He'd started attending counselling which was helping him tremendously. He had, just like me, reached a real low point in his life after the miscarriage and when our IVF treatment didn't work and he had felt like a failure immeasurably. Like many people, he had self-medicated with alcohol, but after a particularly bad night he felt the push to limit his drinking and heal himself, eventually giving up alcohol all together. Talking with his counsellor was very helpful because he was finally ready to do it, he was ready to open up. When we both visited the infertility counsellor after our unsuccessful treatment he hadn't really responded in the way I had, because he simply hadn't been ready to do it, which is why I had attended the majority of the sessions alone. Now he was truly ready and I was so proud of the steps he was taking. It really felt like we were both moving on together. And it cemented that we had made the right decision in not moving forward with adoption at that time.

Chapter Thirteen
Acknowledge, accept, release

I may have found a way to move on, but I still needed to find a place of acceptance. Acceptance was a more difficult thing to achieve, as it meant I had to look at everything that had happened in a wider way, with the benefit of hindsight to aid me. It took me a long time to really look at my life and connect the dots, to really understand that things had happened for a reason. Frustratingly, it isn't necessarily obvious why things happen when they are happening. On reflection it's often possible to identify why something happened the way it did, why you had to live through that experience, and why you didn't get exactly what you wanted. Sometimes 'no' just means 'not now' or 'there's something else for you to do'. Sometimes 'no' means 'change focus and find happiness elsewhere', which is what I decided to do. But it's also something that you have to come to your own conclusion about. It's part of the healing journey; it's part of the journey to acceptance. I may have not been happy about my infertility experience but I was doing my best to accept it and to understand its purpose in my life and the opportunities that arose due to it. And when I really looked at it, so many positives had arisen from the negative.

By 2015, things were substantially better but that didn't mean the same old problems were completely gone and not lurking around somewhere. It didn't mean I would stop dwelling completely or never revisit the past in my mind. As I've said, I believe infertility to be a wound that never completely heals. So when prompted, bitterness and jealousy and unhappy healings can still rise to the surface. I know I'm not alone in feeling this way. It's usually triggered by the same old stuff, like someone announcing their pregnancy with a scan photo on Facebook. Or someone posting the photo of their newborn. Or receiving an invitation to a christening or (the increasingly popular) baby shower. Or being unable to relate to a friend who has recently had a baby because that's all they can talk about and you just have nothing to contribute to the conversation.

I've said it before, it can be difficult. It feels unfair. And it evokes an odd mix of feelings. You're not a horrible person, you're happy for whoever it is. Happy they're having a child and starting a new chapter in their life. But it's a reminder that you're not. You're not getting pregnant. You're not getting to experience motherhood or fatherhood. It's a strange thing to cope with. Feeling happy yet thoroughly gutted at the same time. It's something that impacts you without having any control over it. No matter how well you've moved on, or how happy you feel with your life, that sting still hurts. It also changes friendship dynamics; you might feel lost or that you suddenly don't belong within your friendship group. It doesn't feel great. Sometimes you end up being on the receiving end of an ignorant comment, like, 'Can't you just adopt a baby so that we can talk about our babies together?' And you have no idea what you can possibly say in response because you're blown away by the insensitivity.

And, of course, as any person will know after making the decision to try for a baby, suddenly everyone's pregnant; you see babies or baby bumps everywhere – especially as you get towards a certain age where all your friends decide it is time to grow their families. You may feel you're on the outside looking in at a party you've not been invited to. You don't really know what to say. You've never experienced labour or night time feeds or nappy changes so feel like it's a club you're just not allowed in. It's weird, like being alienated from a place in which you used to feel at home.

No matter how far removed I became, no matter how comfortable I became in the knowledge that my period would come at the end of the cycle, no matter how calm I tried to be about the knowledge that I would never get pregnant, I could still experience that feeling slowly climbing up my sides like nausea.

If you're reading this full of experience and knowledge of infertility or if you've been to the darkest night of your soul and don't know how to get back to the light, please just know it does get better. I know that one of the most frustrating things when you are going through treatment or suffering infertility is when someone tells you 'it gets better'... because you can't actually see beyond your current feelings and 'it gets better' just sounds belittling. But I get it now – it does get better, but only if you're willing to accept that your life might not look how you wanted/planned/wished it to look. It's about trusting the route that life is taking you on. Surrendering and releasing.

I've been there, I've experienced it. I know how it feels abundantly. So how do you get past this? How do you stop feeling like you're some baby-obsessed person? Here is my advice:

Firstly, don't deny yourself these feelings, allow them to be. You need to take care of yourself and show yourself love, understanding and patience.

Secondly, you have to look at your life and be grateful for what you have. This may seem difficult but it's important. Don't ignore all the good and focus only on the bad.

Thirdly, you need to take advantage of the opportunities in life that don't involve children. What do you want to do that doesn't involve getting pregnant? There are many wonderful experiences in life that do not involve having a baby – what are they? Explore what these things are for you.

There are stages in infertility, and the obsession is at its worst in the first couple of years. After a while (or many years, in my case) you do reach a place where you've formed some sort of acceptance (doesn't mean it doesn't get you down now and then though) and you're focused on other life events and experiences.

I know that some people feel that they cannot imagine their life without children, but there are other ways to have children in your life, and when you feel ready, you can explore those options. I know it feels unfair and cruel that so many others fall pregnant and have children (sometimes that they don't even want) and yet you can't, but unfortunately that's what's happened (unfair as it may seem). Widening your goals and dreams to include other things in life will help you.

Finding a focus or a hobby like running or education or travel, or whatever you like to do is so beneficial. Seeking help from a charity or a counsellor or simply a friend that understands can have abundant benefits. It's okay to feel confused and torn and happy and sad and angry all at the same time. Infertility is difficult. Allow yourself to feel how you feel and don't berate yourself. Widen your focus and reassess what you want to achieve in life. You never know when a miracle will occur and you never know what door will open for you. But you have to be open to see it all, otherwise it'll pass you by.

In my case, if I had been fertile and fallen pregnant straight away I would never have lost all that weight, never run marathons, never worked towards fitness qualifications, never started editing, never started writing. You never know where life will take you. The thing with life not responding in the way that you wish is that it ends up throwing all kinds of other opportunities your way – half of which we don't even notice.

However, that did not remove the crippling and damning feelings of failure from my life. No matter how much I've achieved or how many running medals I obtained, the utter failure to reproduce could swallow me up until I kicked and screamed until it spat me out again. Despite attempting to accept my situation the pain still existed and could be evoked because there were reminders everywhere. It's impossible to avoid. Releasing was even harder still – I could accept but how could I release myself from it? The truth is that surrender and release happen organically and in their own time. I couldn't force myself to release myself from the shackles of the past or the weights I dragged along with me beneath the surface just by clicking my fingers. I just had to wait for them to slowly drift away with patience and an open heart.

I was becoming an infertility advocate, keen to use myself as an example of how it does get better, because I felt that the way I'd turned my life around in one year really was a surprise to myself and those around me. Thing is, I thought then and I still think now that it's time we reclaim what life is and where it can take us. Life is so precious that for me or you to waste it feeling sad that we cannot create further lives is veritable tragedy. And it would be lovely for that realisation to have cured me and you of the infertility burden and I know it doesn't, but it can lift us higher.

The knowledge that you and me are worthy and special and can find meaning in our lives without procreating is something to believe in. Because there is so much more out there for all of us, so much we can do and can contribute to the world. Yes, it's lovely to have children and I wouldn't take that joy away from anyone, but if you can't – like I couldn't – there shouldn't be any shame there. We need to remove all shame, all blame, all feelings of failure and unworthiness from infertility. Yes, it really sucks but it really is not the end of the world – mine or yours – even though I know it feels that way time and time again. No man is less of a man because he doesn't make sperm in copious measures, and no woman is less of a woman because her ovaries do not perform as they are biologically expected to.

We are not defined by our fertility, we are not measured by numbers and tests and drugs and procedures. We are beautiful beings who deserve happiness and are able to give happiness to others. Let's count the positives and move forward with those rather than lingering on the negatives and the things we cannot change. We all have things to be grateful for.

Infertility is a very personal and individual journey and I can only speak from my own experience. I can only share how I felt, how I tried to rebuild and how I moved on. Any advice comes from how I lived through it. But there is a way for everyone and it happens in your own time and at your own pace. Be positive and always hold on to hope.

Remember – when it rains look for rainbows, when it's dark look for stars. And when the sky is too dark and all you can see is blackness, just keep going.

Chapter Fourteen
And then it all changed

You know, life is a funny thing. It has surprises in store that you cannot fathom or predict. Here we were, fostering a place of acceptance and peace, and happy with our future plans together, when behind the scenes God had other ideas.

For thirty-one years I was the youngest person in my immediate family, but then my sister-in-law gave birth to a daughter in February 2015 and although we were yet to meet (due to living in different countries) we were thrilled to have a niece and see the family extend. We had also been asked to be godparents of our friends' little girl as well, which was a huge honour, so it felt as though we were finally having children in our lives, even if they weren't our own. My relationship with my husband was doing better than it had in as long as I could remember, and I had another new job, which I was going to do alongside the current one. It was a job that I'd been trying to get for a while.

One day towards the end of March, a couple of weeks after my husband and I had run the Llanelli Half Marathon together, I set out on what I hoped would be an eighteen-mile run – a distance I needed to cover or I was going to get way behind in my marathon training. London was only a month away and I had raised £1065 for charity so far. It was a lovely sunny day with a breeze – good conditions for a long run. Except I felt hot and awkward. I just wasn't enjoying it. I kept stopping to walk. I binge texted a friend so that I could rest. I couldn't believe I had picked up a virus or something. I was down, I thought that at this rate I would need to walk miles and miles in the marathon, as well as in the twenty-mile Llanelli event that was coming up; it was disheartening to say the least. I really wanted to finish quicker this time, or at the very least get through it without hurting myself or becoming ill. So, on that very pretty day, after running/walking about six miles I went home and lay down on the sofa, exhausted.

I was angry to have managed to become so run down so late on in my training. Still, I had my goddaughter's christening to look forward to the next day, so tried not to worry too much. After having a rest I thought more about the failed long run. It wouldn't be the end of the world if I had to walk a little more in London, the atmosphere alone would get me through it. And I had that second marathon in October, which I could step up my training for and finally finish in a time that I had trained for. As the day progressed, aside from tiredness, I didn't detect any other symptoms brewing, so put it down to tiredness from my impending period, as I didn't have a sore throat, cough or anything.

The next morning I woke early. It was one of those occasions where you wake up wide awake with no real reason to. I got up and went into the bathroom, trying not to wake my husband as I went. Without being fully conscious of it, for some reason the following thought occurred to me:

'We still have loads of those cheap strip tests left over from the second IVF attempt – and they expire this month. May as well do three for the hell of it. I'm not due on my period for a couple of days, just do it as some twisted form of fun, they're going to be negative anyway...'

Why I knew that they expired that month, I'm not sure. It didn't seem like something I'd remember. And despite it being a little odd, it did seem like a harmless thing to do. The tests would have to be thrown away anyway, I may as well use them. A pointless thing to do perhaps but in my early morning mental state, it seemed like that right thing to do. So I peed in a cup and dipped three tests. I have no idea why I did three tests. Why not just the one to start? Who knows? I placed them down on the packet and went to put a pot of coffee to brew. When I returned to the tests, a couple of minutes later, I assumed that I would simply look at the negative results and throw them in the bin and just go on with my day as if I hadn't ever so strangely decided to take the tests in the first place. I picked up the tests and scanned them. All three tests had a line. Faint, but unmistakably a line.

My mind started racing. What the fuck was going on? Were they positive? Could they be? Are they defective because they're old? Why had I decided to do these tests out of nowhere? What the fuck was going on?! Why had I made the decision to do this? Who cared that the tests were due to expire? Why did that matter? What the hell was happening?

I went straight upstairs with the three tests in my hand, shaking, and my eyes welled up with confusion and emotion, and woke up my husband, who wasn't too pleased to be woken up so early on a Sunday morning, at least an hour ahead of the alarm clock.

'Look at these tests! Look at them! They're positive – look!'

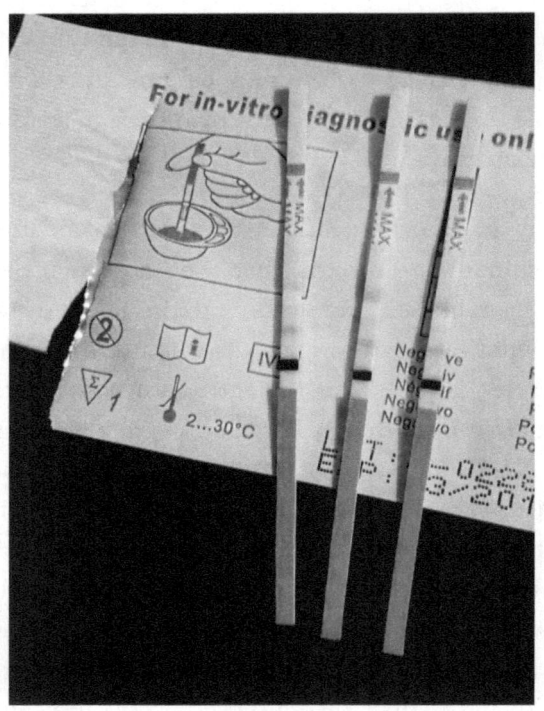

Was this happening now? Now that I'd just got a new job. Now that we had plans for the year. Now that we were finally getting comfortable just being a couple? Had I finally lost my mind and was fabricating a baby? Was I really pregnant?

My husband – in shock – didn't believe the tests. After all, they expired this month, could they be trusted? Doubt re-surfaced in my mind as well. This couldn't be happening, could it? The last time we saw a fertility consultant he basically said my eggs were shit and my husband's sperm were lighthouse attendants. I don't think he knew what to say either, but despite feeling dubious I could tell he was keen to get another test to confirm the result. We agreed we would buy more tests that day, as soon as we could. But it was Sunday. The shops didn't open for hours and we had a long drive and a christening to attend, which we were very much looking forward to. So we got ready as normal. I drove us to Brecon and we stopped in the Morrison's to buy a couple of tests which we agreed I would take when we got home.

Before I'd left the house I'd sent a panicked Facebook message to a friend. I needed her to use a crystal and dowse the question – was I pregnant? Her dowsing would know; I knew it would. Although dowsing was never totally accurate, I just knew it would be today. I don't know why I believed that the dowsing would be correct as dowsing wasn't even something that I personally did! I didn't actually say what was wrong in the message, I just said that I needed to speak to her urgently, and then I spent most of the day near Hay on Wye and had no signal. This caused her unnecessary panic. We had a lovely time and it was just wonderful to become godparents. At some point during the reception after the christening I had enough signal to explain to my friend what was going on and asked her to dowse whether or not I was pregnant as I didn't want to take the new shop-bought test until I got home. Peeing on a stick in a public toilet just didn't seem right (yet using some almost expired tests that morning 'for the hell of it' somehow had done?). She did dowse it but also dowsed whether or not she could or should tell me the outcome and it told her not to tell me. The suspense continued.

The car ride home was never ending. Everything seemed to smell extra strongly and I was tired. We debated waiting to do the test in the morning of the next day, as it would likely be a stronger line if we waited – if it really was true. We finally got home very late in the afternoon and despite all the discussion in the car I knew that I had to do one of the tests straight away. I couldn't wait.

There it was – the second line. A second blue line creating a cross. It wasn't very strong but it was there. I showed my husband but still we weren't totally convinced. After seven years of infertility it would take more than a few faint positives to make us believe it was real. I said that if the test in the morning showed a stronger line then we would know and we would have to trust that result. Surely if five tests were positive then it must be true. I'm unsure how either of us slept that night with so much possibility swirling around our minds.

The thing was, the next day I was due to drive to Bristol very early in the morning and for the entire week to do the next part of my fitness course, the personal training diploma, but now it seemed totally irrelevant and I just wanted to stay home and take time to absorb what was happening. But I didn't have enough time to really think it through. I did the fifth test before embarking on the long drive to Bristol. The test was positive and the line was darker. I showed my husband the test before I left. We had to believe it now.

During that week driving back and forth to Bristol, I don't think I took anything in on the course or quite frankly cared much about it at all, I could barely concentrate on any of it. I was in complete shock and felt like I had no idea what was going on. After the first day of the course I remember walking to the chemist to buy more pregnancy tests and prenatal vitamins. I couldn't fathom if this was real or not. I was in disbelief and extremely anxious.

I was terrified of the following –

1. Perhaps I wasn't pregnant and we'd had a bad batch of tests.
2. Miscarrying again.
3. That I had created the whole thing within my mind and it just

wasn't real.

Over that week the total number of tests increased to sixteen, including some digital tests which made me panic that something was wrong. The number of weeks rested at two to three weeks one day, and the next day one to two weeks, and the day after one to two weeks. I spent so much time googling, panicking that this indicated miscarriage. It reminded me of the tests after that first IVF cycle, the line getting fainter and then it all being over.

Once the course in Bristol was over I visited the doctor and begged for an early scan. I needed something to prove to me that I really was pregnant and that everything was okay. She told me to come back at seven weeks and then they'd be able to contact the early pregnancy unit and explain my situation. She said that with my history they'd more than likely agree. I'd had no bleeding whatsoever, which I took as a good sign and the normal, non-digital tests were getting much stronger, so by the end of that week we finally believed it was happening. But unfortunately I became terrified that something would go wrong.

A couple of weeks later I did two more tests, just for a little bit of extra peace of mind – one digital and one normal. The blue line was so dark I'd never seen anything like it. And the digital test now read three plus weeks so that made me feel more confident. I just needed to be positive now. It was going to be okay. It had happened, it was our time. My husband repeated this to me whenever I became scared. He said he knew all would be well because it was now our time. We'd been through our struggles and this was going to work out.

Of course, this didn't completely calm my anxiety. My mind was working overtime. I was still in complete shock. Passing five weeks was significant to me as it was further than we had got with our pregnancy during our first IVF treatment cycle, then getting to seven weeks felt like a real achievement, so I was hopeful when I attended my doctor's appointment to request the early scan as agreed with the first doctor I saw. It was a different doctor and he told me that I absolutely could not have an early scan. There was no question about it. Despite my history. Despite my anxiety. I had to wait for the twelve-week scan. (Which ended up being at fourteen weeks – tormenting me by making me wait that little bit longer.)

I left that appointment close to tears and once I got to the car I cried. I just needed reassurance, I needed to know that the baby was really there and safe and well. I was frightened. We'd been told by our consultants that we would never achieve a natural pregnancy, so I needed the reassurance that everything was okay. I couldn't cope with anything going wrong. I decided we needed to book a private scan but after discussing with my husband we decided that we would wait. Booking an early scan would be giving in to my anxiety. I had to believe that all was well and stop worrying. If my husband the pessimist believed it would all be okay, then it really must be okay.

One by one, I cancelled all my plans for the year. The first was the London Marathon, second the Bristol and Bath Marathon, and then the half marathons and other events in between I either transferred to my husband or to a friend. I also cancelled any further attendance modules for the fitness course (after an awful experience at an assessment, I swiftly realised that it was not the right time to continue with it. This did nothing to help my general feelings of failure but there wasn't much I could do about it). It was strange to think that I had been really looking forward to all these events and trips away and now it had all been brushed away. I know some people happily continue running and working out when pregnant but I just knew I couldn't. Pregnancy was zapping all my energy and that failed eighteen-mile run the day before I did the first pregnancy tests had really set the tone. I was too tired and too frightened to do anything even remotely strenuous. Funny really to think I was qualified to train ante/postnatal women and yet I couldn't even think of doing any form of exercise (other than walking) myself.

It became the worst kept secret. We didn't announce it on Facebook as we wanted to wait for the scan. But we told lots of people straight away or just whenever we saw them. I even wrote about it on my blog three weeks before the scan as I figured no one I knew personally really read it so no one would notice. And I tweeted. Because I needed to talk about it. I couldn't keep quiet. I was scared but I knew that if something bad did happen I would need to talk about that too. I think it was such a shock to us both that we alternated between being too frightened to talk about it and also being unable to shut up about it. It was a real combination of hope and fear and we were just holding on for the first scan. I remember saying to a friend that my real fear was that the scan would just show an empty uterus and I would be sectioned for imagining a pregnancy. I knew that was just a stupid thought really but having nothing other than the home pregnancy tests to confirm the pregnancy was setting me on edge. I wanted to be excited and to plan life with a baby but I was just too scared to get my hopes up after having so many disappointments in the past. Of course, I had pregnancy symptoms. I had nausea and sickness, I was exhausted, emotional, and everything seemed totally normal. But still, I was terrified of disappointment and further heartbreak.

The first trimester (especially after experiencing infertility) can be a bit of a psychological nightmare, so the weeks in between the first positive test and the first ultrasound can be a bitch. I finally saw the midwife at ten weeks for the booking in appointment. She came to the house and asked a lot of questions, went over options and gave us some information. Now I had a pregnancy file to keep with me and take to all my appointments, so that made things seem a little bit more real. Of course, I worried about that file. What if I lost it or it accidentally caught fire? Would I get in trouble? I don't know if other women have such ridiculous thoughts or whether it's just me. But, still no one had examined me or offered a blood or urine test. It really was all on my say so. And what if I was wrong? What if the tests were all wrong? All eighteen of them.

Eventually the scan date was looming and I couldn't sleep at all the night before the scan. I had played so many different scenarios in my mind before eventually banishing all of them and just thinking about seeing the baby. But I felt sick all morning, I just wanted to get it done. I needed the reassurance I'd been waiting for. When we sat there in the waiting room, my bladder ready to burst with water in preparation for the scan, I had lots of thoughts running through my head again. What if there's something wrong? What if there's just nothing there? What if she does the scan in silence and just said, 'Erm, there's nothing there, why are you wasting our time?' What if she rushes off to get a doctor? What if I accidentally wet myself during the scan due to drinking so much water? I looked around at the other women clutching their pregnancy notes and wondered if they were calm or whether they were full of ridiculous thoughts and panic like I was.

When we were called in, I was shitting myself. Figuratively, not literally. I climbed up onto the bed, flopped out my tummy; she squirted on the jelly stuff and then started the scan. She was silent for about three seconds while getting the positioning correct before pointing at the screen and saying, 'Ah, here's the baby.' A healthy baby was chilling out in my uterus and we could see it there on the screen. I felt tears slide down my face as I watched the screen in awe. That blobby thing on the screen was our baby. We really had done it. It had taken seven years but we really had done it. We were having a baby. My husband held my hand as we continued to watch, it was one of those moments that we will never forget as we never thought we would ever get to experience it, but my husband was right, it really was our time. All the years, all the negative tests, all the injections, all the procedures, all the pounds lost, all the tears shed, all the dark moments, all the hopeful thoughts, all the miles run, it had led to us this moment – seeing our baby for the first time on the ultrasound screen. It was really happening.

The baby wasn't in the position the sonographer wanted for some of the tests so I had to drink more water and walk around for ten minutes before coming back to be re-scanned. Of course, the lazy baby hadn't moved but the technician did the best she could. I really thought I might wet myself at this point. When the scan was done I pretty much ran to the toilet. And we had scan photos. Finally. Finally, it would be us making the Facebook announcement and showing a rather personal view of my uterus to the world. It was our time. I couldn't stop looking at the scan photos as we waited for the sonographer to type up a report for my pregnancy notes and then waited for our appointment with the consultant. I cried again. Out of relief. Out of disbelief. Out of sheer bloody happiness. There really was a baby. I wasn't crazy. There was a baby. And my husband basked in the triumph that his balls did in fact work.

Of course, I was apprehensive about sharing so publicly online because I didn't want to cause anyone who'd experienced infertility or a loss any pain, but we'd just waited so long for this that we couldn't help ourselves. Everyone we knew, knew about our journey and so understood just how miraculous this was. I hoped that if someone had seen the announcement while struggling that it would have filled them with hope and raised their mood rather than lowered it and made them feel upset.

The rest of the pregnancy went by with a mixture of nerves, disbelief and excitement. At our twenty-week scan we found out we were having a girl, which somehow made it all that little bit more real. We finally felt like we could buy baby clothes from that point. Before, I'd felt too unsure of everything to do it. We got her nursery ready in the last few months and I was feeling okay, aside from the perpetual tiredness. Quite often I would feel like I had to pinch myself to check I wasn't asleep because I still couldn't quite believe it had happened. And had happened so out of the blue. I had the words of our old consultant running through my mind, 'fertility fluctuates', and clearly it did. We weren't aware of what had happened to us internally, but my cycle had regulated and ovulation was happening. And the eggs were clearly of a good quality. My husband's sperm count had become normal, maybe even high, and both of these things had happened simultaneously and miraculously, without our knowledge, to bring us the pregnancy my body hadn't produced in seven years. It's a strange thing that we became more fertile in our thirties than we were in our twenties, as it goes against everything we are told by medical professionals. I didn't even fall pregnant at my smallest – I was several pounds heavier when it happened (Christmas weight that I'd forgotten to lose).

But despite all the anxiety and worry during the pregnancy, there were such wonderful moments. Feeling her move in my uterus was such a beautiful experience. One which helped me imagine her as a newborn baby and reminded me that she was there busy growing and developing. I was amazed that I was growing a baby. People kept commenting on how I was carrying a miracle baby, and I knew I was. I knew we'd been blessed with a miracle.

Chapter Fifteen
Re(Birth)

My due date came and went. There was no sign of the baby getting ready to come out. The midwife called around to perform a membrane sweep twice but there was nothing really happening. The consultant decided to book an induction for me at twelve days past my due date. I was really hoping she would turn up naturally before the end of the twelve days but she didn't. So on day twelve I went into hospital to be induced. I was on a ward with two other women, both of whom had been there for a few days already, so this wasn't suggestive of induction being a quick process. I was given a pessary for the first twenty-four hours to see if this would dilate me as upon arrival I was not dilated at all. The pessary looked like a tea bag and had big long strings so you could pull it back out easily when its time was up. It was pretty weird. The other ladies on the ward were chatty so the time went by quite happily. At first it didn't seem like anything was happening with the pessary so I worried that it would be days before anything progressed. I went to sleep that first night praying that it wouldn't take too long.

In the early hours I woke up in pain. I didn't realise I was having contractions as they weren't very long and were every two minutes, so I assumed it was just some pain related to the pessary and the changes taking place to try and bring on labour. Later that morning my husband arrived as soon as he could and I told him that I'd had pain in the night but I still didn't realise the significance and neither did he. When the twenty-four hours were finished I removed the pessary (now affectionately nicknamed 'the pissary' due to the fact that I had peed all over the strings without thinking several times...) and went back to wait for the midwife to check my cervix.

When she arrived she sent all the partners away to the visitor room and she closed all our curtains for privacy. I was last to be seen and as the other ladies weren't dilated enough to have their waters broken, I was sure I would be the same. I didn't mean to eavesdrop, but you couldn't really help overhearing when mere curtains were all that separated you. When she came to examine me I was stunned when she told me that I was four centimetres dilated with regular contractions and was ready to go up to the delivery suite to have my waters broken. It was really happening. I was overwhelmed with emotion and cried when she told me. I told her that it was just because it had taken so long and I felt like labour was never going to happen. She didn't realise that I meant this in a much wider sense, of course, but years of emotions hit me at that point. Really, I'd been waiting eight years to go to the labour suite.

She pulled the orange and peach patterned curtains open and went to make the arrangements. She must have told the partners it was okay to come back to the ward because soon enough all the men were back. I explained to my husband what was going to happen and I'm sure he felt as I did. We packed up my belongings and waited for a new midwife to come and collect us and take us up to the delivery suite.

I was quite nervous as the pain I'd already experienced had been reasonably significant and I didn't really know what to expect next. After we were settled in the delivery room the midwife came to break my waters. She inserted the amnihook up through my cervix to rupture the membranes. The waters trickled out slowly; it certainly wasn't like what I'd seen on television or in films where a clear liquid just gushed out. Once that was done it was just a waiting game: I was at four centimetres and needed to get to ten to push.

One funny moment from the first few hours of labour was the midwife getting annoyed with my husband. He was starving hungry, so went off to the canteen and brought sausage and chips back with him. She was not at all happy but I thought it was quite funny so didn't mind. She kept saying that it was making her hungry and kept asking me if I wanted to make him go and eat his food elsewhere. We spent ages watching the television in the room, but it was hard to concentrate. At one point a late repeat of the Jeremy Kyle show came on but I said it had to go off because it was far too surreal to watch Jeremy Kyle while in labour.

My contractions were slowing down so I was given a hormone drip to help labour progress, and I had gas and air should I need it. At some point in the process, I requested an epidural as the pain was becoming too much to handle and I was exhausted. It wasn't plain sailing from that point onwards, however, because the baby was moving from back-to-back to sideways and was at an awkward angle. The epidural hadn't worked in the way it should have and instead of contractions I was experiencing one constant pain in my back. My husband heard the midwives whispering about a c-section (caesarean section surgery) a couple of times but the doctor who intermittently came in to assess me was adamant that we would continue trying to birth vaginally.

At some point in the early hours of the morning I reached ten centimetres, but then went back to nine centimetres because of the baby's positioning. When the midwife was confident I was going to stay at ten centimetres, pushing finally began. But it was all rather pointless as no matter how many times I attempted to push she wasn't budging, and now my contractions were slowing again and there were no more drugs they could give me to get them going again. The doctor kept suggesting that I lie on my side to encourage the baby to move into a better position but every time we tried this the baby's heart rate would slow, so the situation was starting to become urgent.

We were now into the morning of the next day, fourteen days overdue, and the midwife told me we were going to wait for the changeover of doctors, due to happen at nine o'clock. Almost on the dot the new doctor arrived in my room, I was the first person she saw. I had been in active labour for over eighteen hours at this point. She examined me and heard the details and immediately said that we had to do a c-section straight away. I was scared but relieved because at least the baby would be out and safe, rather than stuck. Suddenly, I was signing consent forms and everyone was hurriedly getting ready for surgery. My husband was putting on protective clothing and one of those stretchy hats.

I was wheeled into the operating theatre and I was amazed at just how many people were present. I'd agreed to let some students observe as well, so it was a full house. There was someone present just to talk to me, which was good because she was very calming. My husband was incredibly anxious but was holding it together for me. The doctor had wanted to top up my epidural for the procedure but I refused – I had already had my epidural topped up twice during labour because it wasn't working enough to mask the then continuous pain, so I had a spinal block instead, which worked. I didn't want to risk having a general anaesthetic should the epidural have proved ineffective. There wasn't anything to do other than lie there and wait for the doctor to cut me open and pull out my baby. There was a big screen in front of me so I was none the wiser to what was happening, other than what I was being told now and then and the odd painless feelings of the surgery.

At twenty-six minutes past ten she was out. And she cried. My husband peered around the screen to see her being lifted up and we both cried at hearing her screaming. I'll never forget hearing her cry and seeing them wheel her by on the way to be cleaned up and weighed. I asked them to lift her so that I could see her face. She was nine pounds exactly. She was then wrapped up she was brought back over and held in front of me on my chest. I kissed her little cheek and couldn't quite believe I was looking at our little girl. She had blonde hair, blue eyes, a squished little red face and head due to her awkward positioning. Here she was, two weeks late, our baby. Her dad then held her while I was being stitched back up. She wouldn't stop crying so he sang Jingle Bells to her. He couldn't think of anything else and it was December after all. Those were magical moments.

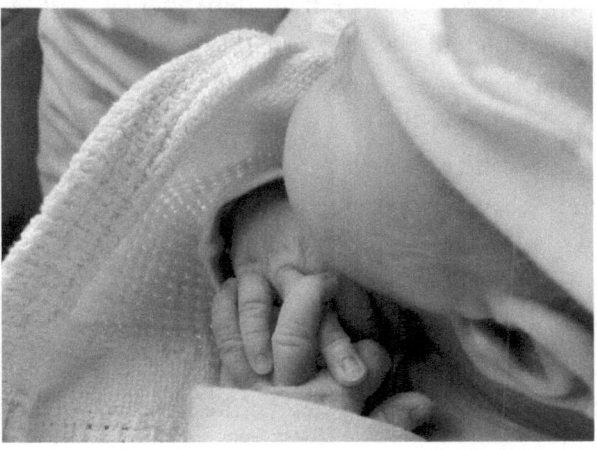

At this point I would love to say that it was all wonderful and amazing with no more issues but I would be lying.

Unfortunately, before we left the theatre I became unwell and this continued for a couple of hours. I was sweating profusely, and vomiting and light-headed. They had no idea why. They just decided it was a vasovagal episode. On reflection I think it was probably a reaction to the various anaesthetics and the trauma of the experience. This meant I couldn't hold my baby and I couldn't try and breastfeed. I was lying down flat watching my husband changing her first nappy and giving her her first bottle. I was watching on in amazement, part of it seemed so surreal but wonderful. The other part of me was jealous and felt useless that I couldn't feed my baby myself.

I wasn't allowed to go to the postnatal ward for hours due to my blood loss, lack of urinary output, and this vasovagal episode I was experiencing. At one point the midwife and health care assistant were brushing my hair (which was soaked from sweat) and tying it up in a bun for me because I couldn't even manage to do it myself. When I was finally able to sit up and hold her, we tried breastfeeding, but nothing really happened. Finally, we were sent to the high dependency postnatal ward, and I was completely overwhelmed, both with love for this nine-pound miracle in front of me and also with everything that had happened during her birth. I remember just watching her sleep in her clear plastic crib next to me and couldn't believe that she was mine. She was so perfect, so brilliant. I was amazed just looking at her. I continued to try and breastfeed but she didn't seem to want to latch so she had formula and I did my best to get her any colostrum I could through pumping. I stayed in hospital for only two nights after her birth, as I kept asking to go home. I was so relieved to leave the hospital. It felt so good to be home.

The community midwife figured out pretty quickly that my daughter had a tongue tie, so that explained the issues with latching and the awful pain when feeding. After her birth I had felt unwell. I was waking up drenched in sweat, and I had a lot of strange pain. I was crying constantly and everything felt too much to handle. The midwife (who was calling daily at this point) did a wound swab and sent it off and we thought little more of it. I assumed how I was feeling was how everyone felt after a c-section and labour. I also had numbness up my right leg, which was being reported to the anaesthetist.

A few days later I was feeling even worse, and we were back at the hospital for my daughter to have her tongue tie sorted so that we could get back on track with the breastfeeding – my milk still hadn't come in despite pumping as well as trying to feed her. As we were at the hospital we called up to the postnatal ward to check on my swab result and to see the anaesthetist. The anaesthetist examined me and said it was just one of those things and that the numbness would go away by itself. As our baby was fine after having tongue tie sorted, and the anaesthetist had set my mind at ease, we were just waiting for the swab result before we could leave. One of the midwives had ushered us into one of the empty wards and said to wait there, we did and didn't think too much of it, assumed they were just going to prescribe some antibiotics and we'd be on our way.

When the next midwife came along she explained that I had a serious infection and needed immediate treatment. I had a raging temperature as well. This was the first of two hospital admissions. The next two weeks pretty much consisted of antibiotics (IV and tablet form) and being in and out of hospital. Breastfeeding was no longer an option because all the medication and time in hospital meant my milk never arrived. I assume that my body was so focused on fighting the infection that it gave up, but she did have about a week of intermittent colostrum. I struggled to accept that I wasn't able to breastfeed her and I felt as if I was already letting her down.

After struggling with infertility for all those years, being unable to breastfeed just felt like another knockback, another failure. But she thrived on the formula, it had got rid of her mild jaundice quickly as well, so it was just something that I had to accept and release, knowing that I had done all I could.

I finally made it out of the hospital for good on Christmas Eve. Just in time to experience our first Christmas together as a family of three. And despite being totally out of it, I still really appreciated the wonderful time we had together. I had spent so much time dreaming and wishing for moments like this and now we were finally experiencing them.

Only really as we approached her reaching one month old did I start to feel more normal, but in truth it was months before I properly recovered from the c-section and subsequent infections. The first few weeks were a blur. Looking back now, I wish I hadn't given myself such a hard time about everything. One thing I learnt about being a mother is that you have to let go of how you think it'll be and accept how it is. I was worried about everything all the time and I would have doubts about my ability to cope and give her everything she needed while I was still healing.

The thing was, after over seven years of infertility, two unsuccessful IVF treatment cycles and getting pregnant naturally out of the blue, I really had expected everything to be practically blissful after all we had been through. When you've wanted and waited for something for so long you build up so many expectations around it. The pregnancy was anxiety-filled, her birth traumatic, and the immediate aftermath was so difficult.

But you know what? It doesn't matter. I would do it all again to have her, step by step. Having a baby is a lot of hard work and sleep deprivation, but also so much wonder and love. She was the most amazing and beautiful being and we loved her so much. She was who we'd been waiting for. We were lucky, we finally had our miracle.

Chapter Sixteen
Becoming a mother

As it took me a long time to recover from the birth and infections, I felt as though it took me a long time to adjust to motherhood, which shocked me. But there was a settling in period and a healing period which needed to happen. And there was joy. Lots and lots of joy and love to fill each day.

Having children after a long period of infertility puts you into a strange world. It's like your success is tinged with guilt because of thinking of all the people who are suffering like you used to. Like being the lucky one makes you feel bad for those who aren't as lucky. When my baby was three months old it was Mother's Day. My first Mother's Day. I felt wracked with guilt for most of the day. Instead of enjoying the fact that I was now a mother and had this amazing baby, all I could think about was all the people out there who were still trying or who'd had to accept that it would never happen, just like we'd had to. I just found myself feeling awkward about it, as if I couldn't really enjoy the day properly because I was so acutely aware that Mother's Day is such a sad day for many, including myself not so long ago.

In particular I was conscious of those suffering from infertility. The women (and men) out there that wished they could feel special on a day like Mother's Day but instead it just highlighted the pain and sadness that they tried to ignore. Seeing photos and cards and comments on Facebook was lovely, yet they could evoke a conflicting feeling inside, being both happy for your friends/family and also terribly sad because no one is wishing you a happy Mother's Day/Father's Day as well. The frustration of not knowing if it'll ever be your turn can be overwhelming, and it's heart breaking to finally accept that it never will.

Infertility can feel like a heavy weight you carry around, weighing you down. It can feel even heavier on a day like Mother's Day. I tweeted that morning about how I felt and a friend replied and told me to enjoy it and reminded me that I'd waited years for this day. She was right. I couldn't let remembering the sadness ruin my first Mother's Day. But I could send love and prayers out to those who needed them with the hopeful promise that whether they became parents or not, there would be good times ahead for them.

I was taking photos of her each month to chart her growth and it was astonishing to see how quickly she was becoming her own little person. Even by three months she had changed so much. We had her christened in a little chapel in rural Pembrokeshire one Sunday; my stepfather performed the service for us. It was a dry but wintry March day and in a way it felt a bit unreal. During the service I found myself get a little bit choked up because I was there christening my own child, not someone else's. I wasn't just a member of the congregation today, I was up at the front holding my own daughter. So many times I'd had little daydreams about having my potential baby christened but that had been something I'd had to let go of after IVF had failed. Now there I was holding my baby, standing by her father, watching her gain godparents and meet a load of family and friends that she hadn't seen before and it was like seeing everything anew through her eyes. Although it was quite a normal and common occasion, to me this was the stuff of dreams and wishes which I never thought would come true.

There were lots of things that under normal circumstances wouldn't be quite so significant or thought provoking, but I was constantly finding myself connecting back to things from the past and being moved by how much things had changed. Even taking her for her injections at the doctor's surgery made me think back to when I worked in a surgery and would be aware of baby clinic going on downstairs, or even assisting with the admin as it was happening, and feeling bitter or jealous watching mothers come and go with their little ones. Wondering how they'd all managed to achieve this one thing that I couldn't. Of course, I had no real idea if it had been easy or a struggle for those mothers, but my natural assumption at the start had been that everyone else had had an easy time and I hadn't. I quickly and acutely learnt that so many people had suffered from fertility issues and there were many dreams and miracles walking through the doors of the surgery every day, as well as those that had turned up almost instantaneously.

I was also totally thrown by how a song or a film or a storyline on a television show now had a different meaning for me. In particular, there was a song called *Little Something* by Above & Beyond, on their album *We Are All We Need*. I started listening to the CD in January 2015 on my long commutes to work. Typically, when you first hear a new song you don't necessarily consider the lyrics too closely, but after a couple of listens I realised that it was about what your children mean to you. So despite thinking that song was beautiful, I would skip the track. Because when I really listened to this song it evoked past feelings of heartbreak.

Little Something

I wasn't going to be able to have a child and I had to accept it. It was unsettling, but it was part of my mourning at the time. It probably helped me release the emotions I was suppressing. The song would take me back and cause momentary reliving of the past, as music has the power to do.

Fast forward two months to our positive pregnancy tests, and now I was listening to *Little Something* again, but this time it was bringing up different emotions. Excitement and fear. After all those years of infertility I was finally pregnant and I was terrified and anxious that something might go wrong. I cautiously imagined what this little something I was carrying would be like. I was experiencing something totally new with this song – it was following me into this complete change of life. I affectionately started to refer to her as our little something. Finally, when she was born at the end of the year, I was listening to this song again but appreciating it in a completely different way. Again I was moved to tears but my reasons had changed. As I held our little miracle I realised the lyrics couldn't be more apt. Funny how in the space of one year one song can move you for totally different reasons. It just shows how quickly life can change.

That was something that stuck with me. Life really does change quickly and you cannot predict exactly what will happen or when, you've just got to trust that whatever happens is right for you.

I was living a different life now. Once one of heartbreak and trying to find new ways to find meaning, I was now in a place of more calm acceptance. I knew that I needed to trust God more, that I needed to trust my journey more. Back when we initially set the intention to have children, we didn't expect it to take so many years and have so many ups and downs along the way, but the destination was the same place, we just had to take many detours before the timing was right. And believe me, when this is happening and your hope is dwindling, it's almost impossible so see the bigger picture, but the bigger picture is always there, we just need to wait for the clarity which will enable us to see it.

Chapter Seventeen
New life

Once I had physically healed and adjusted to my new life as the mother of a beautiful daughter, I started exercising and trying to regain my hobbies again. Most mornings I would take my daughter out in the buggy and go for a run/walk along the coastal path. After a trip to London for the Running Awards with a close friend and then watching the London Marathon on the TV, the desire to start running again really took hold.

I think that part of me thought it would be easy and the fitness and stamina would just return, as if I had just put them on hold. Wishful thinking, of course. In reality, running again was harder than it ever had been. I was carrying extra weight after the pregnancy and my fitness levels were depleted, so even one mile felt like a mini marathon. Nevertheless, I kept going, kept trying, and slowly I was able to run a full mile. I eventually made it to four miles but with significant walking breaks. I managed to run/walk a 5k and a 10k with a friend that summer – the Newport Kolor Dash and the Llanelli 10k. I really wanted to be a positive example for my daughter. I had thoughts about doing a half marathon in the autumn but I knew that it was too soon for something like that. I knew I had to take it slowly and I wasn't sure if I wanted to train for that many miles either. I didn't have any childcare in place and my daughter would lose patience with being in the buggy if we went over three miles, so 5k was the right distance to focus on at that time.

My daughter's first year of life was quite eventful for enumerate reasons, one of which being my parents' separation. Though it was obvious that things had not been right for a long time, it had now come to a head and separation leading to divorce was imminent. Despite having experienced divorce as a very young child when my mother and father's relationship had broken down, I really couldn't remember much of the process itself, so being so aware of my mother and stepfather's situation was a whole new experience. I remember just feeling so powerless about the situation, and the realisation that I could do nothing to help was confounding and confusing.

It was especially concerning because now mine and my husband's elderly parents were all living alone and all in different places. I found the stress of this situation too much to deal with at times. Going through divorce as a child and then as an adult are quite different experiences. No matter how old you are, if the family you've always known splits apart it's bound to cause tremors. But my daughter had to be my first priority, so I prayed for a healthy resolution for my parents and tried not to focus upon the negativity or get drawn into drama. Life goes on, and regardless of what happens the sun still rises and sets every day.

It's very true that life with a child changes your priorities, and when something's not right you take steps to fix it because you've got more than just yourself to think of. My husband had been seeing a counsellor and then a psychologist to work through his mental health issues and this was going well for him. He was really facing old demons and finding a way out, finding more positive ways to deal with things. We knew he'd been suffering with depression and anxiety, something I'd also experienced over the years, but the psychologist had realised that there was more behind this problem, and that the root cause wasn't purely low mood. He was assessed by the adult autism team and we discovered that he had what used to be referred to as Asperger syndrome – a term which is no longer used for diagnosis. All new diagnoses are simply of Autism Spectrum Disorder (ASD).

Our daughter was about nine months old when we had the official diagnosis from the team and this came as a partial shock and partial relief to us both. My husband and I have always been total opposites, from our appearances to our personalities, so there was a lot that we had just accepted about each other without really considering that there was actually a neurological difference at play. My husband had always worked very hard. He always had a job and had worked his way up to being a financial advisor after graduating university. He also had a Master's degree in Philosophy and many financial qualifications. It's just that his brain was wired differently to a neurotypical person and that caused him to see the world differently, process information differently and struggle with communication. It changed nothing about our relationship other than learning more about our neurological differences so that we could move forward and understand each other better. He remained the dedicated husband and father he always had been.

There was a grieving process for both of us, which is a normal part of dealing with such a diagnosis. Just like with infertility, we decided to be open about his diagnosis. And just like infertility we were faced with varying levels of response from the good – 'he hasn't changed, he's the same person', to the bloody awful. One comment in particular that was extremely inappropriate was being told that now he was autistic we shouldn't have any more children. This came from someone close to us, someone who knew him well. It made no sense. After all, he hadn't suddenly become an autistic person, he quite simply always had been. It was alarming how derogatory the comments and suggestions were from certain people, all sourced from ignorance. He hadn't changed, he was the same caring, loving, educated and hard-working person, but he was just neurologically different and always had been. Really it was refreshing to discover this, not awful to discover it, but nevertheless there was an element of shock for my husband and me to overcome. I remember being particularly caught off guard by that particular nasty comment, however, because despite the ridiculous and insulting suggestion, we had no idea if we could even have any more children. Our daughter was an absolute miracle, so we couldn't know if any more would come to us. We had no plans to try and get pregnant again because we just didn't know if it was an option or not.

Of course, life works in funny and mysterious ways, and unknown to all of us, the moment I was hearing that inappropriate comment a second miracle was busy implanting and developing in my uterus.

Dealing with the diagnosis in one way seemed to be more about managing other people's ignorance rather than dealing with earth shattering news ourselves, and after the initial jolt we were calm. We educated ourselves more on Asperger syndrome/ASD and did our best to educate others when required. Nothing in our day-to-day lives really changed, just more understanding developed. I was happy to stay at home and look after our daughter and my husband was happy to work and support our family. He had his own personal acceptance and reflection to experience, and he knew who he was in a way he hadn't before. He could finally find a personal peace and understand why he saw things differently to other people. If he hadn't felt prompted to address his issues and seek counselling (prompted by our failed IVF treatment) before our daughter was born, he would never have experienced this epiphany or opportunity for such personal growth and understanding.

Unfortunately, the traumatic birth and aftermath had caused me to experience a period of postnatal depression and anxiety, which I'd found very difficult. I took medication for a short time to help. But I was managing this without too much issue now. I think the worry and anxiety before her birth had just taken on an accumulative effect and needed time and patience to lift. I'd have bad and good days, but overall I was focusing more on the present and looking inside myself for answers, rather than leaning on external things. Certain things still got to me, I still struggled with feelings of failure and sometimes would find myself revisiting those sinking feelings. Getting pregnant and having a child didn't remove those feelings in their entirety, they were still there, and I had to work hard not to focus on them. Spending my time with my daughter and watching her grow and develop new skills was such a blessing and gift and she was the light to fill any darkness.

When my maternity leave ended I decided not to go back to either of the jobs I held previously but instead started working freelance as an editor again, from home. This suited our dynamic better. I was especially glad of this decision when one weekend in the autumn I started to have this strange inkling that I was pregnant again. After doing several tests it was clear that I was. Cue another shock, especially since there was only one occasion of no contraception in the entire cycle. So now we had gone from seven years of no contraception before getting pregnant to one single occasion of no contraception and we were pregnant. The universe really does have a sense of humour. I worked out the due date and we would have an eighteen-month age gap between the two children. I know some people might think that even one occasion with no contraception was a silly risk for someone who had only had a baby nine months ago, but given our history, all those years with nothing happening, we didn't even give that one occasion a second thought. We really were being blessed with miracles.

I felt calmer during the start of the second miracle pregnancy than I had done the first time. It was less of a shock and more of a surprise. I was focused on my daughter so it led to less mind wandering and less time to think about negative things. At around eleven weeks I suffered a bleed out of nowhere, but we were able to have an emergency scan that day to check that the baby was okay, and happily all was well. We saw a little twitchy baby on the screen, seemingly happy, so the bleed was written off as a random occurrence. Our scheduled twelve-week scan (which took place closer to thirteen weeks) showed again that all was well, so we breathed easier. We now felt confident to tell everyone. Someone told me that she always thought it would happen like this for us. It seemed that even when we had given up hope that our fertility might change, other people still believed that our children would come to us – and in quick succession.

When my daughter turned one year old, we held a little party for her at our house. I thought a lot about the first year of her life and while it had been a lot of hard work, I couldn't help but feel full of love and belief in the right timing. My little rainbow had taken her first steps and was becoming a toddler, a little girl with her own personality, her own dreams and wishes. Her blonde hair had changed to red and one of her blue eyes had a streak of brown, present from when she was very tiny. It was magical to have brought such a beautiful soul into the world.

At our twenty-week scan for our second miracle, again all looked fine, and we discovered that we were expecting a boy. We were overjoyed for our daughter to be having a little brother. I'd had less inclination this time as to the baby's sex but a part of me deep down had thought it would be a boy because back during our IVF treatment I had secretly felt that the treatment would bring boy/girl twins to us. Of course, it didn't, but somehow that feeling had stayed within me somewhere and it was coming to fruition through a set of totally different circumstances. I couldn't help but feel immensely blessed as we walked away from the hospital after that scan. I prayed with all my heart for health and happiness for us all. Life really had taken us where we always wanted to go, it just had its own opinion on the route and the timing.

At twenty-five weeks pregnant with our second miracle, I was sitting in the waiting room at the doctor's surgery, waiting for the midwife to sign a form for me. The waiting room was reasonably small and there were only a few people in there, none of whom were talking. I noticed two other pregnant women sitting near me and tried to guess how far along they were just to pass the time. The pregnant woman closest to me was called in to see the midwife and then a new patient walked in the door. He seemed to know everyone so spent a while saying hello to the other people waiting before taking a seat on the bench with the remaining pregnant woman. As it was silent in there, it was not possible to avoid overhearing their conversation.

Man: You alright?

Pregnant woman: Yeah just waiting to see the midwife.

Man (surprised): The midwife?

Pregnant woman: Yes, I'm pregnant again.

Man: Oh, well, many congratulations!

Pregnant woman: I'm gutted.

Man: What?

Pregnant woman: I've got three already. I didn't want another one. But it's there now so what can I do? I'm gutted about it.

Man: Do you know if it's a girl or a boy?

Pregnant woman: No, we'll find out next week at the scan.

Man: Oh right.

Pregnant woman sighs sadly.

My mind was working overtime while I was hearing this conversation take place. Part of me was annoyed and part of me felt bad for her. I had no idea what it felt like to have an unwanted accidental pregnancy. I couldn't judge her feelings about her situation because I hadn't experienced her life. I didn't know what it felt like to not go through infertility, and to not wait years to be blessed with children. I didn't know how it felt to decide that you didn't want any more children and then to accidentally become pregnant again. I didn't know how it felt to feel nothing but despair when looking at a positive pregnancy test. I didn't know any other route to motherhood other than my own.

But I do know how I would have felt if I had heard her conversation back when we were trying unsuccessfully or going through treatment or trying to move on and focus on a childless life. Hearing that conversation would have felt like a massive kick in the gut. It would have felt like I was being mocked. Here's a woman so fertile that she's now on her fourth child and she doesn't even want it, and there I would be feeling barren and jealous and upset. The one thing I wanted and couldn't achieve, she could easily achieve and so flippantly not even be happy about it or want it. It would have stayed with me and found its way into my thoughts when I was feeling low. It would have been there tormenting me, making me feel like a failure as a human. Why should she get pregnant with children she doesn't even want and I not get pregnant with a child that I so desperately desire? The unfairness of it all would have been overwhelming.

But, of course, I wasn't hearing it as an infertile woman. I was hearing it as a mother with her one-year-old daughter in the buggy in front of her and a second child busy growing in her womb. I wasn't sure what to think about her words. Part of me felt that old hurt from infertility rise up, consumed with the injustice of the situation and the awfulness of the woman being unhappy to be having another baby, but the other part of me just felt sad. I didn't know what it must have felt like to be unhappy about a baby, I didn't know if that woman was suffering with antenatal depression or some other problem. I didn't know if she felt she could cope with a fourth child or not. I didn't know what her home life was like. I could never judge her now like I could have so easily before.

I still believe that all babies are miracles and are brought to your life for a reason, because you are the right parent for that child, but I can't overlook the fact that sometimes things just don't work out well. Mental health, addiction, horrible living situations, and other circumstances beyond the basic mother and child connection can be at play. A thought came into my head while overhearing the conversation: 'Once she sees her child after giving birth all her doubts and fears will be gone.' And perhaps that's all it really was – the woman was scared. Scared that she couldn't handle another child. Scared she couldn't cope with another birth. Just scared. We all get scared.

But it was a big reminder to never judge another person as despite how things look or despite what people seemingly carelessly say, no one has any idea what dwells beneath the surface.

I placed one hand on my bump and my other hand stroked my daughter's face and I could have cried with happiness then and there. I could see that I had been blessed with miracles. I could see that everything that had happened previously had led up to this new life, this new family. None of the tantrums or broken sleep mattered compared to how I felt inside. I'm not sure I have the words to describe just how grateful I am to have been given these gifts and to have experienced such love. This was what I'd always wanted and I prayed for other couples suffering with infertility to achieve their happiness, whether from being given the baby they'd been waiting for or finding peace and happiness in their lives in other ways. Happiness is always possible and miracles happen every day in all sorts of wonderful ways.

Believe in yourself. Trust yourself. Love yourself.

Chapter Eighteen
Motherhood is a strange beast

The twisty path of life often ties me in knots. Sometimes I feel sure that I know where the path is leading only for the direction to change, leaving me confused but in awe. I gave up on the dream of having children for it then to be made reality. Head spinning with disbelief, another positive pregnancy test showed me that there were still more twists that needed to untwine. And in a short space of time there were two babies in a home where there once were none.

I was adamant that I would never have another c-section. As soon as I knew I was pregnant again, I immediately wanted a VBAC (vaginal birth after caesarean). I told my consultant during our first appointment that I didn't want an elective c-section and I know he was pleased about this as they like to encourage vaginal births if appropriate. It was agreed and it was all looking good until a late scan showed that the baby was breech... bugger. My first baby was transverse until very late on and now this one was upside down. They gave me until almost 38 weeks for him to turn, which he did. Brilliant. I actually remember the moment he turned around. It was the night before the scan and

I was standing in the doorway of my bedroom experiencing the oddest feeling of the pregnancy so far. I wasn't sure if he was trying to burst out or what. The scan confirmed that he was now head down, so all I had to do was wait to go into labour. Wait to go into labour – something that only happened due to induction drugs the first time. I don't know whether I am just awkward as arse or what, but my body doesn't seem to ever want to go into labour naturally. I kept waiting for contractions to start or my water to break, but not even a hint of labour was happening. I'd had some Braxton Hicks contractions earlier in the pregnancy but they seemed to have dried up now. At my term appointment with a different consultant she examined me and performed a quick scan. All of a sudden my VBAC was off the table. He was a very big baby and he was too high up. He wasn't engaging. I was booked in for my c-section for the next working day and I was left to sulk. I longed to go into labour naturally. It really didn't help that we were having very warm summer weather, so combine a heavily pregnant woman with a heatwave and it's not pretty.

Off we went on the Monday morning for my last minute elective c-section, already drenched in sweat before leaving the house, leaving my daughter with my friend, and trying not to be scared. I felt immense guilt at leaving my daughter, even though I knew she'd have a fun time with her faerie godmother. This was all a false start, however, as we were sent home later that day and told to return the next. Too many c-sections were booked in for the same day and I was the last one booked so the first one moved. Tuesday morning stank of déjà vu but once we got to the hospital things were better as I was first on the list this time. I know I shouldn't have felt this way about having a c-section – giving birth in any way should have just filled me with joy because not so long ago it was a dream which had become so distant that it was never going to happen – but I was hormonal and hugely pregnant, so I was indulgent. It was such a different build up compared to my previous experience. The first time round, with my daughter, I was taken from the labour suite, exhausted and drained from the induction and long labour straight into the operating theatre and barely had any idea what was going on – I was only pushing a second ago, wasn't I? This time I was totally 'sober'. I was happy that I would be meeting my son that day, but I was terrified of the surgery. And after going through all the admin involved and then walking to the operating theatre, I burst into tears while having my spinal done. Not because it was painful, but because reality was hitting and I was frightened. The procedure and the aftermath were weighing heavy on my brain. Still, it felt bloody embarrassing.

I don't know if everyone experiences the blood pressure drop after the spinal at the start of surgery, but I do and I swear it makes me feel like I'm dying. And then comes the nausea and vomiting, continued dizziness, etc. But otherwise I was ok and just trying to focus on the baby, not the procedure. When it's all happening it's the strangest thing because you're awake, staring either at the ceiling, or your partner, or the sheet in front of your face, and down the other end people are cutting you open and birthing your baby for you. My son was born, safe, well, and crying – although had to be dragged out with the aid of forceps. I had a quick glance at him before looking on as my husband and the midwife took him over to be checked and weighed and all that stuff. Watching my husband's pure happiness was quite magical. So many thoughts ran through my head but one I distinctly remember was feeling so grateful that my husband was such a good father. I also wondered what my daughter would make of her brother. My husband came over to tell me that our son was 10lb 6.5oz, and I thought he was joking. I'd thought my daughter was big enough at 9lb. Our boy was brought over and held in front of me and I kissed his cheek. He immediately stopped crying. Truly a wonderful moment that I will never forget. There's nothing quite like the first time you see or hold your baby. Suddenly the tiny human that you've spent nine months growing and imagining is presented to you and your whole being just floods with love. He was super cute, but not chubby, just long and generally big.

My husband held him for the rest of the surgery, which was going on a long time now. Apparently there was a lot of scar tissue and damage from the infection last time to tidy up. But it was going on so long that I started to feel the pain of it all. Apparently my placenta was 'ragged' so I was having IV antibiotics because of that as well.

I held my son as we were taken back to the ward, which was wonderful because I didn't get to hold my daughter for a long while after she was born. Then I threw up everywhere. Twice.

All the while, I'm overwhelmed with love. I'm looking at my son's little face and all the worrying about the surgery, all of the worrying about looking after a baby and a toddler whilst recovering from surgery, is gone. I know I'll cope. With love I can do anything.

The aftermath (recovery period is probably a better term) was better, but I don't think that would be difficult to achieve considering how bad it was the first time. I managed to get some odd swelling and an infection (nothing serious), but otherwise I was ok. I had anaemia again and was suffering with postpartum migraines, but they seemed a fair trade to have such a beautiful boy.

I'll still never understand why people think c-sections are an easy option because in my experience they are bloody hard (maybe I'm just crap at c-sections?). I don't think there is such a thing as an easy birth. Pregnancy and childbirth are not easy. And neither way of getting a baby out of your body is ever pain free. If I'm totally honest, I did feel a little bit gutted that I will (probably) never experience a vaginal birth, but there was zero point in dwelling on this. The method of delivery is irrelevant, the baby at the end of it all is that counts, and the baby is worth everything. When I looked into his big blue eyes, utterly bewildered of this strange world he'd just entered, I felt true innocence and unblemished possibility. This baby, my son, such a beautiful little soul. He had dark hair, like me, but not for long, as it soon fell out and grew back blond.

A baby, a child, a human, is such a precious thing. We must always, always know our worth and believe in ourselves to the depth of our beings. Allow it to flood our bodies from the tips of our toes to the tops of our heads. We must love ourselves. As we are.

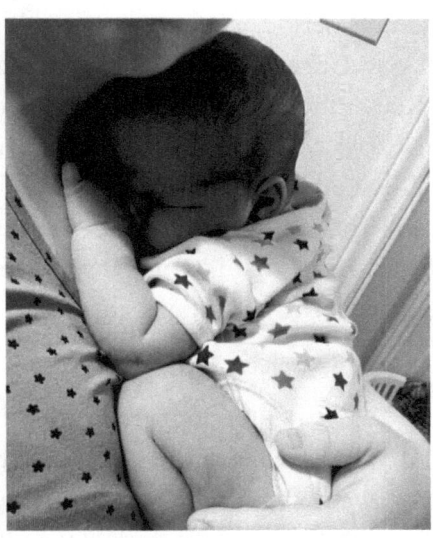

A lot of things were easier second time round, from breastfeeding to sleep, and in the early weeks of my son's newborn days I thought I had escaped postnatal depression, but it was there, again, lurking, ready to knock me over. Along with the anxiety. I went through phases of shutting myself off and deleting my social media accounts. I went on antidepressants again only to stop taking them a week later. I found little things could totally knock me off course – a mean comment on social media, or bit of extended family drama – those things were shattering to me. When you've written a book about your extremely personal journey you have days when you feel totally exposed and vulnerable and want to delete the book from existence, but then those moments pass and you remember why you've done it. You remember that there's a chance it may help someone, somewhere.

After all the positivity I've gained and all the focus on the good, the negativity can sweep in and I don't even realise it's there until it's got its feet up in front of the fire. Depression and anxiety hang around and wait for the moment to turn up and ruin your life for an indefinite period of time. Anxiety loves it. It waits for you to feel good, feel better and then smacks you across the face again. Remember me? I'm still here. I revisit the tools I learnt back in the days of struggling to cope with infertility and I cuddle my children and smile at their laughter, but sometimes nothing will help. And in those moments the best advice is to just keep going and know that it won't always feel like this. The postnatal fog did again lift, and things got easier, but some days remain difficult.

Experiencing postnatal depression after infertility was a real shock to me. I'd wanted children for such a long time, and I finally had what I wanted. So why was this happening to me? It was as if I thought my previous infertility experience would shield me from any problems post birth, but I realise this was nothing more than wishful thinking. Postnatal depression can affect anyone and it's no one's fault. The important thing is to seek help. And be kind to yourself always.

I've spoken at length about how people asking questions about whether you want children or not can be tremendously difficult to receive, and now as a mum of two I sometimes get asked whether or not I want a third (as if such a thing would be in my control), and it's made me realise that the inappropriate questions never end. There's always something. And really, truly, a question is only hurtful because of the significance we place on the subject matter. I was having a conversation with a friend of mine about this and she didn't think she'd ever been asked when she was having children, but then after further thought she realised that she had been asked a few times, but, the question didn't have much significance for her because she didn't want children. But our significance is our own and our triggers are our own and no one needs to apologise for any of it.

Falling pregnant nine months after my daughter's birth seemed to invite inappropriate questions.

Was the pregnancy planned?

Was this one an accident?

Was he the product of a boozy evening?

Erm... I don't really feel like giving you information about my sex life right now, if that's ok? It's funny how brazen people can be. And is there such thing as an accident after seven years of infertility?

Having two children with an 18-month age gap meant I needed

a double buggy. This buggy always seemed to act like a magnet for people to comment. Usually something like: 'Ooh you've got your hands full!' To which I would smile, say yes I do, and go on my merry old way. But every now and then I'd get a strange remark. I was walking around the supermarket one day, pushing the two children in the double buggy and a man stopped me. He said the usual 'Ooh you've got your hands full here!' and then he looked at me and said:

Are they both yours?

I was confused but told him they were. What was he expecting me to say?

No, I rent the ginger one.

No, I just saw the smaller one the side of the road and brought him with me?

No, I stole them both.

No, I operate a 'I'll take your children to the supermarket with me' service, because taking children to the supermarket is just so much fun…

Unaware of the strangeness of his question, he smiled and went over to the potatoes.

Another time, my daughter and I were walking down a street near to where we live. I was holding her hand and we were doing a slow toddler walk. An elderly couple stopped us and said hello.

Woman: My grandson is ginger too. We don't know where he gets it from.

I smiled and nodded.

Motherhood is a strange beast

Man, pointing at my daughter: He's like a little Ed Sheeran, isn't he?

Me (paused with a 'what on earth do I say to that' awkward smile): Hah... yes.

I couldn't bear to see the look on their faces by telling them my little Ed Sheeran was actually Edwina Sheeran. And no offence meant to Ed at all, but the red hair is where the facial similarities end.

Where there are people, there will be inappropriate comments and awkwardness.

Motherhood is a strange beast. Everyone seems to have an opinion on what you're doing, but all the opinions are entirely contradictory. You often feel like you just cannot win because when you decide to do one thing (breast, bottle, co sleeping, not co sleeping, nappies, cloth nappies, etc.) there's always another side telling you that you're wrong — at least it feels that way. It's an incredibly hard job and I think it would be nicer all round if people supported each other rather than just condemning people for differing opinions. Shouldn't we lift people up rather than tear them down?

The craziness of life continues on. The balance of a baby and a toddler remains a delicate balance, but then there's nothing more magical than that curious moment where happiness is palpable. When I turned 34, I decided to act upon a closely guarded goal that I had been harbouring since getting pregnant with my daughter – I decided to go back to university and do a part-time psychology degree. I find it provides me with a good balance while staying home with my children. I love learning new things.

To my shock, the 'baby weight' didn't just fall off, and it's been a struggle to shift each pound. And that too has fed my failure complex. I was embarrassed that as a 'champion' of weight loss I had managed to gain weight and not lose it immediately. As much as I know, as much as I've learnt, that feeling of being a failure is never far from my door. So, again, I needed to learn to love myself as I am and know that I'm ok as I am. I would love to lose some weight for my health, but I have to accept that it'll take a little longer than I am used to. I'm slowly re-introducing structured exercise back into my routine. The health benefits are too great to ignore.

Since having my son, I've thought a lot about the early miscarriage I experienced during that first IVF cycle. I assume it's because having two children close in age reminds me of twins. I'm reminded of all the possibility and all the wishes and dreams I sent out to the universe, which were all shattered when I lost the two embryos so early on. I never really allowed myself to mark their due date or think about how old they would be now, because before I was blessed with my children, I found it too difficult to deal with. I didn't really want to think about my one chance of children that had slipped away all too easily. I couldn't find a way with dealing with being on the brink of everything, only to have it swept away with the tide. The waves would just keep crashing. I will always carry the memory of those two little souls with me just as I will never forget my infertility journey. All the dreaming, wishing, waiting, IVF treatment and heartbreak will always be with me. It has been a massive part of my life. I cannot express the gratitude I feel to have a daughter and son, and for being their mother. Looking after them is the greatest honour I have ever received. They are total opposites already, but both wonderful and special in their own unique ways. And I pray every day that they have happy, healthy lives filled with positivity and love.

The rain will always be there, tapping against the window, but we wait, patiently or impatiently, and one day we will see that rainbow – that symbol of our blessings, or the symbol of how we are moving on positively with our lives – and our hearts will be fit to burst.

At the end of each day, when we lay down to sleep, when we think about the mundane moments of the day, and dream the big dreams of our futures, all that really matters is love.

CHAPTER NINETEEN
Why I believe in miracles

People mention miracles fairly frequently. It's either a massive, unattainable thing 'it'll be a miracle for that to happen' or it's mentioned nonchalantly 'it was a miracle I caught that train'. But miracles really are out there and occur all the time, it's only our perception of them that illuminates or diminishes their exposure.

Quite often I think we need to experience a big miracle in order for us to get that jolt to wake up. For me it was getting pregnant with my daughter. She was the big miracle that shed light on all the unrecognised miracles that had preceded her arrival. As a result I am more open to recognising a miracle, no matter how small. I truly believe that any pregnancy is a miracle, every person is a miracle, and that life in itself is miraculous.

In writing this book I wanted to help others who may be struggling with infertility or with life in general. I don't have all the answers but I know that sometimes what we seek is just not ready for us. Sometimes it's simply the wrong time. I prayed for IVF to work, for us to very specifically get pregnant (with twins) from our IVF treatment. But the answer was no. Because that wasn't how it was meant to be for us. I had things to learn from the process, things to grieve and things to gain. While I understood the answer to be a resounding 'no' at the time, really it was just 'not yet'.

Infertility and hitting rock bottom really showed me that there was no one I needed to be other than myself. We all have different faces that we show to different people but all that matters are our true selves. I started to care less what people thought about me. If I wanted to wear hot pink Doctor Martens I was going to. Because we are all so valuable to the world, but as ourselves, not as the person we think the world wants us to be or to look like.

The greatest peace comes from being yourself and loving who that person is. That's where miracles grow. That's where life begins. We've all heard the saying – 'life begins at the end of your comfort zone', but it's true. I showed the world my vulnerable self when our IVF treatment failed and I was rewarded with gifts. Without realising it at the time, telling my story helped other people who were struggling. It made them feel not alone and in turn did the same for me.

Quite often, especially with social media, there's a temptation to only show our best selves, to make our lives look perfect, harmonious and desirable, but when you strip back the façade and let people know who you are, tell people your experiences, you're creating real strength in your vulnerability. I found my greatest strength in the most testing of times. Sometimes I'd write a blog post and feel like I was sharing too much but then I'd receive a message from someone who was also struggling and I realised that my experiences could help someone else move on and find peace. Finding the positives in a difficult situation isn't easy. I can't pretend it is easy.

When my world shattered around me after that second IVF cycle it took my faith with it, it drained the positivity from my life, but I worked hard to regain it. After everything failed I saw two roads in front of me, self-medicating with alcohol and food or rebuilding by running and working towards the marathon. Working towards something, something which would provide focus. It was difficult to get myself out of bed at dawn to get outside and run, it was hard to see the point, see the justification. But I still did it. I still rebuilt rather than just allowing further destruction.

I'm certainly not saying that anyone needs to run a marathon in order to recover, this is too extreme a suggestion. Not everyone wants or needs to run such an event, but finding something to take hold of your interest and allow you to move forward positively is essential. This could be anything – it is all down to an individual's preferences and abilities. The important thing is rebuilding rather than causing further destruction. When things fall down we pick them back up, not leave them in the gutter. Small gestures go a long way to healing yourself. Just taking the time to focus on something you can do to move forward will have such far reaching benefits that you cannot even imagine. It proves a commitment to yourself and your healing.

Losing weight after a lifetime of obesity was a miracle. Finding the strength to run a marathon was a miracle. My husband finally seeking help and finding out he had Asperger syndrome after a lifetime of struggling was a miracle. Getting pregnant after all that time and failed treatment really was a miracle, and falling pregnant so easily a second time was equally so. I had no idea these miracles were waiting for us, so I had to find a way to move on with life and when I did everything changed. Miracles don't necessarily come to you in the way you expect them and then when they do, it may not be exactly how you expected it, but

Little Something

what is life without surprises?

I think back a lot to when the counsellor told me about the analogy of people appearing normal but being weighed down by all the life expectations they carried with them below the surface. In truth, there really isn't anything that we need to do other than take care of our basic human needs. There's no need to turn yourself into a superhuman who is good at everything they do and succeeds at everything they try. There is just the need to find happiness in whatever way, shape or form you can. There's a reason people tell you to be kind to everyone you meet. It's because no one knows what personal battle they are facing, no one knows what dwells below the surface.

I think back to all the avenues I went down which all led to dead ends or I just decided it wasn't right for me – teaching, fertility treatment, various courses, and various jobs. Each one of those things, whilst they did not provide what I expected them to, all contributed to my life journey, all provided learning opportunities and unseen connections to other possibilities.

There are no real failures, just life experiences. Infertility is not a failure, not having the career of your dreams is not a failure, not having whatever it is that you want is not a failure. They are opportunities of a different sort, a prompt to assess your life and decide what you really want, what really makes you happy and finding a way to overcome the sadness and hurt. You never know when your time is waiting for you and you never know exactly how you're going to get there. Don't worry about how, just focus on what you want and if it's right for you, you will get there.

Those expectations that dwell below the surface are like weights dragging you down. Cut the cords and fly. Find release in your own time, through your own way. Focus on love, on gratitude, your blessings, but most of all, believe in yourself.

Miracles happen when you least expect them. They grow out of the darkest of times and take you on journeys you could have never predicted or expected. And that is the beauty and wonder of life.

Bibliography

Helpful websites:
Fertility Network UK
www.fertilitynetworkuk.org

Fertility Friends
www.fertilityfriends.co.uk

Miscarriage Association
www.miscarriageassociation.org.uk

Adoption UK
www.adoptionuk.org

Mind: For Better Mental Health
www.mind.org.uk

Anxiety UK
www.anxietyuk.org.uk

PND and Me
www.pndandme.co.uk

PANDAS Foundation: Pre and Post Natal Depression Advice and Support
www.pandasfoundation.org.uk

Cry-sis
www.cry-sis.org.uk

Samaritans
www.samaritans.org

The National Autistic Society
www.autism.org.uk

Verity: PCOS Charity
www.verity-pcos.org.uk

Infertility, pregnancy and birth:
WHO: Infertility Definitions and Terminology
www.who.int/reproductivehealth/topics/infertility/definitions/en/

Infertility
www.nhs.uk/conditions/infertility/Pages/Introduction.aspx

Definition and Prevalence of Subfertility and Infertility
www.ncbi.nlm.nih.gov/pubmed/15802321

Diagnosis and Fertility Tests
www.nhs.uk/conditions/infertility/pages/diagnosis.aspx

Infertility Procedures and Treatment
www.nhs.uk/Conditions/Infertility/Pages/treatment.aspx

Induction of Labour
www.nhs.uk/conditions/pregnancy-and-baby/pages/induction-labour.aspx

Caesarean Section Surgery
www.nhs.uk/Conditions/caesarean-section/Pages/introduction.aspx

BabyCentre
www.babycentre.co.uk

Weight loss, fitness and running events:
Body Mass Index (BMI)

www.nhs.uk/chq/Pages/3215.aspx

Weight Watchers
www.weightwatchers.com/uk

Cardiff Half Marathon
www.cardiffhalfmarathon.co.uk

Llanelli Half Marathon
www.llanellihalf.co.uk

Swansea Half Marathon
www.swanseahalfmarathon.co.uk

Yeovil Half Marathon
www.yeovilhalf.com

Brighton Half Marathon
www.brightonhalfmarathon.com

Bristol Half Marathon
www.runbristol.com

HBA 5-10-20
www.hba51020.org

Beast of Bryn
www.bwystfilybryn.btck.co.uk

London Marathon
www.virginmoneylondonmarathon.com

The Wales Marathon
www.thewalesmarathon.com

Bristol and Bath Marathon
www.bristolbathmarathon.com

Race for Life
raceforlife.cancerresearchuk.org

Llanelli/Sospan 10k
www.sospanroadrunners.co.uk

Newport Kolor Dash
www.stdavidshospicecare.org/event-details/kolor-dash

The Running Awards
www.therunningawards.com

VRUK running club
www.veganrunners.org.uk

Fundraising:
The Children's Trust
www.thechildrenstrust.org.uk

MACS
www.macs.org.uk

The John Hartson Foundation
www.johnhartsonfoundation.co.uk

Barnardo's
www.barnardos.org.uk

Cats Protection
www.cats.org.uk

Cancer Research UK
www.cancerresearchuk.org

Other:

Geraint Richards
www.geraintrichards.wales

Above & Beyond
www.aboveandbeyond.nu

Above & Beyond: We Are All We Need album
store.anjunabeats.com/collections/above-beyond/products/above-beyond-we-are-all-we-need-cd-1

Jillian Michaels
www.jillianmichaels.com

Michelle Gordon
www.michellegordon.co.uk

Acknowledgements

I have to start with expressing immense gratitude to Paul, Tabitha and Dominic. This is as much their story as it is mine and I could not have written it without them. Thank you to Paul for allowing me to share his personal experiences without reservation. Thank you to Tabitha and Dominic, and Tabitha's morning nap. If it weren't for them, I wouldn't have written this book. And if Tabitha didn't have a morning nap, I definitely wouldn't have.

I'm very grateful that my friendship and working relationship with Michelle Gordon spans many, many years. She's been a constant support and wonderful friend, and this book wouldn't have been brought to publication without her. Thank you for your editorial, creative and technical help and advice, encouragement and awesomeness. Big thanks to Laura Wilce for your editorial help and advice. I'm so thankful we were placed next to each other in our university accommodation all those years ago. Laura has been there through light and dark and always willing to talk about nothing and indulge in inappropriate humour. Cheers to Amanda Caton, Alex Watts and Liz Gordon for your help and advice during the publication process.

And finally thank you to the family, friends, co-workers and strangers who have made a difference, whether they know it or not.

About the Author

Elizabeth Lockwood was born in a small town in South Wales, but grew up all over the place. She spent most of her childhood listening to music or trying to be the funny one. She gained three English degrees at different universities and tried (but mostly failed at) several types of career. Elizabeth followed a rather manic path to motherhood. After years of infertility, weight loss and marathons, the ups and downs have taken her from heartbreak to happiness and helped her become a more positive person.

Elizabeth lives in Wales with her husband and children. She loves keeping fit, studying psychology, editing books, listening to ABGT, writing, and anything magical.

Elizabeth's website can be found at
www.elizabethlockwood.co.uk.

www.ingramcontent.com/pod-product-compliance
Lightning Source LLC
Chambersburg PA
CBHW030332230426
43661CB00032B/1383/J